# The Handbook to Home Health Therapy Documentation

CINDY KRAFFT, PT, MS

HCPro
a division of BLR

*The Handbook to Home Health Therapy Documentation is* published by HCPro, a division of BLR.

 5 4 3 2 1

Download the additional materials of this book at *www.hcpro.com/downloads/12514*

ISBN: 978-1-68308-073-2



HCPro provides information resources for the healthcare industry.

HCPro is not affiliated in any way with The Joint Commission, which owns the JCAHO and Joint Commission trademarks.

Cindy Krafft, PT, MS, Author
Tami Swartz, Editor
Erin Callahan, Vice President, Product Development & Content Strategy
Elizabeth Petersen, Executive Vice President, Healthcare
Matt Sharpe, Senior Content Production Manager
Vincent Skyers, Design Services Director
Vicki McMahan, Sr. Graphic Designer
Sheryl Boutin, Layout/Graphic Design
Phillip Couch, Cover Designer

Advice given is general. Readers should consult professional counsel for specific legal, ethical, or clinical questions.

Arrangements can be made for quantity discounts. For more information, contact:

HCPro
100 Winners Circle Suite 300
Brentwood, TN 37027
Telephone: 800-650-6787 or 781-639-1872
Fax: 800-785-9212
*Email: customerservice@hcpro.com*

*Visit HCPro online at www.hcpro.com and www.hcmarketplace.com*

# Contents

Supplemental materials can be found at *www.hcpro.com/downloads/12514*

 

# About the Author

## Cindy Krafft, PT, MS

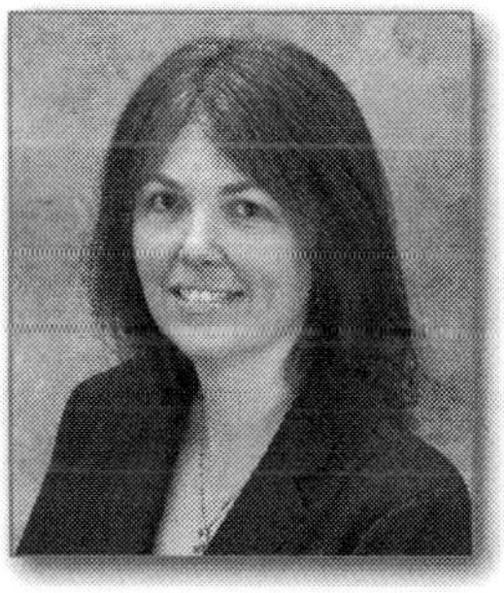

**Cindy Krafft PT, MS, HCS-O,** brings more than 20 years of home health expertise that ranges from direct patient care to operational and management issues. Years spent in the homes of patients proved to Cindy that this was the best setting in which to focus on functionality and the specific challenges faced by each patient. Providing care in the home environment is different than any other setting, which is clearly evident in both training and consultation activities.

For the past 15 years, Cindy has been a nationally recognized educator in the areas of documentation, regulation, therapy utilization, and OASIS. She has served in several national projects as well as an expert resource for OASIS updates. She focuses on providing the knowledge and tools to operationalize external requirements while keeping the needs of each home heatlh the driver of care. Cindy has been involved at the senior leadership level for the Home Health Section of the American Physical Therapy Association and is its immediate Past President. She works with APTA and CMS to clarify regulatory expectations and addresses proposed payment methodologies to ensure the long-term participation of therapy services in home health. She has written two books, *The How-to Guide to Therapy Documentation* and *An Interdisciplinary Approach to Home Care*, and co-authored her third, *The Post-Acute Care Guide to Maintenance Therapy.*

Contact Cindy Krafft at *krafft@valuebeyondthevisit.com.*

Chapter 1

# Welcome to the World of Home Health

Many therapists have had little or no exposure to home health as part of their education. Once they accept a position with an agency or contract company, they may become frustrated because they do not understand the unique expectations that surround this area of practice. The documentation challenges in this setting are significant, and there have been limited sources of information to guide the home health therapist in meeting the demands of payer sources and agencies—until now.

## Home Health PPS

Prior to 2000, Medicare paid home health agencies on a per-visit basis. There was a set dollar amount for each discipline, and as long as "skilled" issues were present, care could continue unabated. In order to gather standardized and consistent data, The Centers for Medicare & Medicaid Services (CMS) created the Outcome and Assessment Information Set (OASIS) instrument, with nationwide implementation in agencies effective January 1, 2000. The tool focuses on outcome measurement, as the name implies, but it was selected for a secondary purpose as well: Because every agency in the country was going to use it, CMS decided to use some of the questions to determine what payment would be made for the care provided. Thus, the relationship between the number of therapy visits and reimbursement was born. References to Medicare may appear a narrow focus at first glance, but the key concepts apply to home health regardless of the payment source.

Along with OASIS came the model of the 60-day episode for home health. As long as patients qualified for services, they were allowed to continue those services, but formal reassessments were now expected if care was going to extend beyond 60 days. Essentially, the industry was placed on a budget, with OASIS used to calculate the dollar amount associated with each individual patient, and the Home Health Prospective Payment System (HHPPS) era began.

## 'Fixing' Therapy Documentation

It wouldn't take much effort to simply create a list of words or phrases that therapists could use to improve their documentation. Although some have tried this route, they've had only limited success, because content tends to become repetitive quickly and lacks both patient specificity and a clear picture of therapist involvement. Therefore, before getting into the details of documentation content, it is important for therapists to get a broader perspective on this unique practice setting, to understand the "why" behind the expectations, and to empower them with a working knowledge of how to document the necessary information clearly.

## Time to Make a Choice

Some might argue that therapists' practice decisions were never influenced by the reimbursement model. This argument is true in the majority of agencies, which consider the patient's needs to be the driving force for decision-making. Nevertheless, therapists struggle with documentation and how it affects reimbursement. Therapists know that patients need their services, but they often feel overwhelmed and frustrated with getting these services written down on paper or into a computer. In desperation, they say, "Just tell me what you want me to put down."

The time has come to change how therapy documentation and care delivery are viewed in the home health setting. Therapists must take back control of their documentation, with a clear orientation on how to create meaningful content efficiently while keeping the focus on the patient. At the end of the day, the patient is the primary reason that any therapist stays in the home health setting, and they must embrace effective documentation as a critical element of excellent patient care.

 

Chapter 2

# Documentation: The 'D' Word

People generally choose to enter healthcare professions based on their desire to help others. Regardless of practice setting, documentation is often seen as a necessary evil. Any discussion of documentation tends to provoke feelings of frustration as well as the assumption that high-quality content requires a large volume of detail and time. In order to better understand these concerns, consider how therapists learn to document the care that they provide.

## Documentation in Home Health

### *Documentation tools*

There are issues with documentation tools no matter what the format. Thus, gaps in documentation cannot be blamed on any specific tool: The responsibility for providing documentation that clearly supports medical necessity falls squarely on the shoulders of therapists. Each therapist must be diligent in creating appropriate detail that is a balance of "check boxes" and narrative content to show each patient's individuality.

### *Completing documentation*

A frequent strategy for managing paperwork in home health is to defer documentation until the end of the day or the following day. Doing so can allow therapists to be home at a reasonable time and be available for personal events. On its face, this plan seems like a good one, but it raises questions about the accuracy of the information being recorded. Meaningful key details can be lost between care delivery and the time that the note is generated, especially when multiple visits have occurred in the interim. As an example, think about the first person you encountered yesterday: Can you provide a detailed description of what that person was wearing, his or her hair and eye color, and the first words spoken? Without a plan to remember all of that information, some aspects of the description are likely to be omitted. Jotting down a few cues to refer to later is a good way to ensure accuracy and clarity.

## Making Peace

No one would suggest that documentation is delightful and that therapists will learn to love it, but therapists must reach some level of acceptance in order to move past the current environment of confusing and conflicting information that is leading to content that is insufficient to support medical necessity. High quality in assessments, visit notes, and clinical summaries is not about the amount of information they contain but rather about the focus of the content. Mythical lists of the correct statements to use to ensure payment are not the answer. The level of detail needed to support the ongoing inclusion of physical therapy, occupational therapy, and speech-language pathology as integral parts of home health care requires that therapists reclaim ownership of this important issue and revisit what they know to be skilled care.

 

# Chapter 3

# Medical Necessity

One of the largest myths about therapy documentation is that progress equals skilled care. On the contrary, therapists must demonstrate skill—not just progress—to support medical necessity.

The term "medical necessity" is used often in healthcare but can lack clarity for the individual clinician. To clarify, consider the dictionary definition of the word "necessity," which contains a very helpful piece of the puzzle: indispensability. The medical condition can set the stage, but the key element for medical necessity is to define what the specific discipline—physical therapy, occupational therapy, or speech-language pathology—is going to provide to the patient that will have a meaningful impact. Progress in the traditional sense may occur because of these interventions, but it alone will not show skill.

## Looking at It a Different Way

Here is another way to think about it: Imagine that you wake up and head to the bathroom to get ready for the day, and you find that water is all over the floor. It is not a little puddle—it is enough that you know something is wrong. You have to get to work and already have a busy day planned, so you have little time to deal with this situation. You call a plumber and ask him to come over during the day to fix the problem. (For the sake of this example, you are not secretly a plumber or particularly handy in this regard.) At the end of yet another hectic day of seeing patients, you arrive home and go straight to the bathroom. Happily, there is no longer any water on the floor, indicating that progress has occurred. The situation has improved compared to what it was in the morning. On the counter, there is a slip of paper representing the bill for the services provided. It reads: "It was broken. I am a plumber and I fixed it. Total cost is $1,500."

There is little that would make anyone excited about paying $1,500 for anything, but there is also clearly not enough information in the note to justify the amount. Key items are missing, including what the problem actually was, how long the plumber was there working on it, what parts were involved, and what had to be done to install them. Bottom line, you would want to see enough detail to indicate that you could not have taken care of the problem yourself for a lot less cost. At an even more basic level, how do you know that the plumber did not just mop up the water and leave? It would be very disheartening to realize that you paid someone to do a job that did not actually require a specific set of skills.

Connecting this example to documentation in healthcare, why do nurses and therapists continue to submit notes that essentially read, "The patient was sick. I visited him. He is better now. Here is the bill"? The missing pieces are similar: The therapist must show more than the end result of the care and must be clear about what skilled interventions were used to achieve those goals. If you would not accept less from a plumber in your home, why do we expect less from ourselves when documenting the care we provide?

An extension of the progress myth is the idea that a plateau means that the patient has to be discharged. Some agencies have created practice patterns around this idea. They state that if progress is not seen in three visits, then the patient must be discharged, as he or she no longer requires skilled care. However, the lack of progress is not the main factor in deciding to discontinue a skilled service. Rather, the decision to discharge is driven by the determination that there is nothing left for the specific discipline to contribute in terms of interventions that will benefit the patient. The idea that a patient can make clearly measurable improvements on every single visit is not realistic for the patient population we serve. Still, the belief that progress justifies skilled care may be the reason that therapy notes often appear to include arbitrary gains in ambulation of 5–10 feet or in repetitions of exercises on every visit.

In contrast, viewing medical necessity from the standpoint of indispensability highlights the importance of detailed interventions in conjunction with progress, all of which supports the inclusion of therapy services in the plan of care. When analyzing the typical course of care, plateaus happen periodically over the entire episode. Skilled care continues regardless because therapists expect that improvements will happen over time as more skills are taught or as more techniques are applied to this specific patient situation by each discipline involved.

 

## Maintenance Therapy

Any discussion of medically necessary therapy must include the topic of maintenance therapy. Updates to the Home Health PPS have drawn attention to this issue, and there has been some confusion and misunderstanding about how this concept fits into this practice setting. The end result has been the belief that maintenance therapy is a "new" area of growth for home health agencies and that Medicare has expanded coverage, neither of which is accurate. The definition of skilled therapy applies here as well, as it must be clear that the skills of a therapist are indispensible to the patient.

Delivery of therapy in the home setting falls into two general categories, and both are defined by their focus, as can be seen in the following table (Table 3.1). Restorative therapy is based on the intention to see improvements in the patient's functional status as a result of skilled interventions. Keep in mind how improvement is measured, as this is not a "progress is equal to skilled care" discussion. The changes in the patient would impact the quality and/or quantity of functional performance in ways that are meaningful to the patient and that reflect his or her participation in the plan of care. Maintenance therapy, on the other hand, is used in situations where the assessment of the patient situation indicates that substantial improvements are not expected and that the focus is on preventing decline. The plan of care is created with the intention of turning follow-through over to a nonskilled person, like a family member or paid caregiver.

**FIGURE 3.1** **Restorative and Maintenance Therapy**

| ***Restorative Therapy*** | ***Maintenance Therapy*** |
|---|---|
| • Intent is to <u>improve</u> the patient's ability to function | • Intent is to <u>prevent</u> further loss of function |
| • Qualified therapist establishes the plan of care and completes the required reassessments | • Qualified therapist establishes the plan of care and completes the required reassessments |
| • Therapy assistants CAN provide care | • Therapy assistants CANNOT provide care |

 

There are two different situations that meet the criteria of covered maintenance therapy in home health:

> **Situation #1:** It is determined that the patient is not going to show significant improvement and would not meet the intent of restorative therapy. The patient requires the skills of a therapist to make this determination, establish the necessary program, train the appropriate caregiver(s), and make any modifications to the program as indicated. Given the level of skill needed for all of these tasks, only a physical therapist, an occupational therapist, or a speech-language pathologist can perform these visits—therapist assistants cannot participate in the plan of care. In the language of the Medicare manual, covered maintenance therapy would "require the specialized skills, knowledge, and judgment of the qualified therapist to design or establish a safe and effective maintenance program."
>
> > **Example A:** A 68-year-old female with long-standing heart failure is referred to occupational therapy to address her limited ability to perform bathing and dressing safely. The occupational therapist completes the initial assessment and determines that the patient is currently performing these tasks at the same level that she has for the past three years, but the therapist is concerned that she may decline if she does not stay active in self-care. Her daughter is very helpful—sometimes too helpful—and needs to know how to best assist her mom without facilitating additional dependence. The occupational therapist puts together a plan to educate the daughter and initiate a set of activities to keep the patient involved in her own care. After a few visits, the occupational therapist is confident that the patient and daughter have mastered the program and discharges them with the instructions to keep working on the tasks and strategies that were taught.
> >
> > **Example B:** An 85-year-old male with peripheral vascular disease is referred to physical therapy with concerns regarding his ability to safely get up from his chair and ambulate. The physical therapist assesses the patient and determines that his potential for significant improvement is low. The therapist initiates a plan of care focused on teaching the patient and his wife strategies to decrease the difficulty of the transfer by increasing the height of the seating surface and by instituting a daily walking program to prevent further decline. The physical therapist completes several visits to focus on education around these issues and to assess the patient's ability to tolerate a walking program. Once these tasks are

 

mastered, the physical therapist discharges the patient and instructs him and his wife to walk in the apartment complex at least once each day.

**Situation #2:** It is determined that the patient is not going to show significant improvement and would not meet the intent of restorative therapy. The patient requires the skills of a therapist to make this determination, establish the necessary program, train the appropriate caregiver(s), and make any modifications to the program as indicated. The complexity of the patient and/or the program being implemented indicates that it would not be safe to turn the care over to a non-therapist. Based on that determination, a therapist would deliver the maintenance program, as there would be the need for ongoing assessments and modifications to the program based on the patient's condition. This level of complexity indicates that the physical therapist, the occupational therapist, or the speech-language pathologist must perform all visits—therapy assistants cannot participate in the plan of care. In addition to the language of the Medicare manual noted for Situation #1, the following is taken into consideration here: "The unique clinical conditions of a patient may require the specialized skills of a qualified therapist to perform a safe and effective maintenance program."

**Example C:** A 72-year-old female with a history of a stroke three years ago is referred to speech therapy due to concerns over her ability to safely handle thin liquids. The speech-language pathologist determines during the assessment that the patient has been using thickener as ordered but that increased fatigue from her recent open heart surgery has affected her ability to swallow consistently. The speech-language pathologist is concerned that the patient's new caregiver is having trouble remembering how to correctly cue and monitor the patient, and she establishes a plan of care to see the patient to monitor her thickener use and confirm the ability of the caregiver to assist. In a few weeks, the speech-language pathologist is confident that the patient is managing well and discharges her on her original diet, now confident that the caregiver is able to follow through correctly.

**Example D:** A 50-year-old female with multiple sclerosis is referred to physical therapy to assess functional status after a recent hospitalization. Changes in her medication while in the hospital have affected her ability to safely ambulate the limited distance she is capable of to get from her bedroom to the patio. She currently completes that distance, but the physical therapist determines that her ability to do so depends on the timing of her

> medication, which the nurse informs him is still being adjusted. There is a competent caregiver, but the physical therapist knows that he will have to monitor this patient closely and adjust his recommended activities based on her overall status for the time being. Once the medication issues stabilize, so do the patient's functional abilities, and the physical therapist is now comfortable turning over follow-through to the caregiver and discharges the patient.

It is clear that the medical necessity component of maintenance therapy is the need for a skilled therapist to assess the patient, establish the plan of care, train the caregiver(s), and determine when his or her own care is no longer indispensable. The care itself can be delivered and covered when the complexity of the patient or program means that a therapist must be involved. Once again, skilled need is based on the nature of the interventions and the level of assessment and reassessment required by the patient. Maintenance therapy is not covered when the therapist is no longer contributing anything meaningful to the plan of care, as visits have become repetitive in nature and there is no variation in the interventions being used.

Therapists may struggle internally with discharging patients who they know are not going to follow through on recommendations or who will not do the exercises unless someone comes and tells them to. They know that it is very likely that the patient will decline and a new referral may be made. Logic would indicate that simply keeping this patient on service would be better than discharging, but the Medicare benefit does not cover that as medically necessary therapy, as there is no need for the specific skills of a therapist for that level of care.

## Defining Skilled Care

Therapists have spent far too long looking to external sources to define what skilled physical therapy, occupational therapy, and speech-language pathology should look like and how they should be documented. In the actual regulatory language, providing a definition of skilled care is often deferred to the disciplines themselves. Over time, when concerns arise about clarity, payer sources begin to try to drive documentation expectations that derive from the respective professions themselves. For those reasons, therapists need to take a long look at their own disciplines and define as a group what constitutes skilled care, as well as the documentation content that best supports medical necessity.

 

# Chapter 4

# Impact on Therapy Practice

The topic of therapy documentation in home health cannot overlook the role and influence of the Outcome Assessment Information Set (OASIS). Very few, if any, clinicians will volunteer to complete this document, and some have become quite good at avoiding it. The general consensus is that the tool is "extra" work and completed for the benefit of Medicare, with little or no direct use to the clinician trying to care for people in need. A critical element of home health since 2000, OASIS remains an object of frustration and confusion and is in many ways disconnected from therapy documentation.

## Data Collection

OASIS items were developed with the intention of being discipline neutral. That being said, each discipline brings different expertise to the data collection and can have different reactions to and levels of comfort with the individual items. These differences have led to the idea that there are "therapy" OASIS items—namely, the functional areas such as ambulation, transfers, and bathing. However, even though a certain level of skill in these areas is a natural extension of what therapists typically examine when assessing patients, that fact does not limit data collection in these areas to therapists.

At times, OASIS items regarding wounds, dyspnea, and incontinence have been thought of as "nursing" questions, but in reality, they are within the therapist's scope as well. The overriding theme of OASIS is to collect accurate information about a patient in order to determine what changes have occurred over time as a result of specific interventions, which is the core of delivering high-quality care in any setting. Thus, every discipline involved in home health has a stake in showing positive patient outcomes in OASIS.

## Who Can Complete Data Collection

The ability to show the impact of care begins with an accurate assessment at the beginning of the episode. According to the Medicare *Conditions of Participation* (*CoP* 484.55), "A registered nurse must conduct an initial assessment visit to determine the immediate care and support needs of the patient; and, for Medicare patients, to determine eligibility for the Medicare home health benefit, including homebound status." In cases that include nursing and therapy services, the registered nurse is required to complete the admission visit regardless of patient diagnosis or staffing availability. *CoP* 484.55 goes on to add, "When rehabilitation therapy service (speech language pathology, physical therapy, or occupational therapy) is the only service ordered by the physician, and if the need for that service establishes program eligibility, the initial assessment visit may be made by the appropriate rehabilitation skilled professional."

For Medicare patients, the physical therapist or the speech-language pathologist can complete the initial assessment, inclusive of OASIS, when there are no nursing orders present. The need for occupational therapy alone does not meet the criteria for a qualifying service and means that occupational therapists may not admit a Medicare patient to home health. However, they may be able to do so with other payer sources, so each one should be verified independently with respect to coverage criteria. Nursing and any of the three therapies can complete a Discharge, Transfer, Resumption of Care, or Recertification OASIS, and there is no hierarchy of which one can do it. Therapist assistants are not able to complete the document itself, but they can provide valuable insights into the patient's abilities when they understand the importance of the tool.

## Therapists and the Start of Care Assessment

There has been much discussion and debate about the ability of a therapist to complete a Start of Care assessment. Some deem certain components of this task, such as the drug regimen review, skin assessment, and incontinence, as not actual therapy. Although these areas are not traditionally seen as therapy tasks in home health, this unique setting challenges therapists to understand that they are treating entire patients, not isolated joints or specific problems in a vacuum.

Therapists must keep in mind that the task here is to screen the patient to determine whether and when other services are warranted and whether those services are within the scope of a therapist. It is understandable for agencies to decide not to have therapists complete admissions based on limited staff availability, but it is concerning when the decision is made based on a perception that they are not capable of completing that level of assessment.

Therapists must be clear as to the difference between a true scope of practice issue and a task that a specific therapist is not comfortable with completing or competent to complete. Scope of practice is defined by regulation, whereas personal competence is the result of training and experience. Consider this example: Would it be legal for a licensed nurse in your state to draw blood? In the legal sense, it would be accepted practice. Still, would you allow any random licensed nurse in your state to draw blood from you? Probably not. You would want a nurse who is capable and who knows how to draw blood well based on his or her level of experience. The same logic applies to some of the tasks that OASIS requires a therapist to complete: Can a licensed therapist conduct a thorough skin assessment in your state? It is within the scope of practice. Are you as a therapist comfortable and competent completing a skin assessment? If not, then the issue becomes how you will go about gaining knowledge and practice. With any of these areas, it is the responsibility of the professional to know the specific details in the scope of practice document for the state in which he or she practices to ensure that expectations are within the scope of each discipline.

## Collaboration for Improved Accuracy

Agencies must abide by certain regulations in order to participate in the Medicare program, as well as abiding by any state or local regulations that apply. It is important to understand that OASIS is a document with a single signature attesting to the accuracy of the information collected. Combining the home health regulations with the OASIS requirements has led to the widely held perception that the OASIS is the responsibility of one clinician alone, but it is not.

Consider that the *OASIS Guidance Manual* confirms that, on admission, there is a five-day window in which the clinician is able to collect information about the patient. This is the opportunity for all members of the care team involved with the patient to collaborate in order to ensure the highest possible level of data accuracy. It also demonstrates that the whole interdisciplinary team is responsible for participation in OASIS data collection, regardless of who actually completes the document.

The majority of agencies have a review process for the OASIS document to ensure that data collection is accurate. There may be an entire department of people who spend their days reading OASIS documentation. Clinicians have learned to be apprehensive of these staff members, as a call from them means that something is "wrong" and has to be corrected. Busy clinicians may become so overwhelmed with corrections that they no longer care about providing an accurate response and simply want to know which responses will make the reviewer happy. When clinicians show a pattern of inaccuracy, many agencies will refer them for additional OASIS training, repeatedly spending a considerable amount of time and financial resources trying to help clinicians to "get it."

There is another option to consider—collaboration between clinicians who have seen the patient within the first five days since the start of care. This approach requires that all of those involved have a working knowledge of OASIS data collection, regardless of which specific discipline will complete the tool itself.

No one is suggesting that the five-day window should be used in every case. In addition, the five-day window is not about how much time a clinician has to fill out the tool completely. Rather, it is about having the opportunity to go back and conduct additional data collection as the admitting clinician or to seek insights from others.

Note the use of the term "collaboration," which indicates that it is not acceptable practice to carve the OASIS tool into parts and have different disciplines complete sections independent of each other. Many of the frustrations with OASIS data collection are rooted in the larger issues facing home health: collaboration, communication, and documentation.

## Incorporating OASIS Into Therapy Documentation

OASIS influence should extend beyond completion of the actual tool. It includes many important pieces of information that are relevant on all patient assessments. With nursing services conducting the majority of home health admissions in many agencies, the initial contact a nurse has with a patient more often than not involves OASIS as part of the comprehensive assessment. In light of the fact that occupational therapists are not completing admissions to home health for Medicare patients, these evaluations can be disconnected from OASIS and appear very discipline-specific, leaving important broader issues undocumented—such as the presence of incontinence or a current pressure ulcer.

 

Additionally, although speech-language pathologists are able to admit Medicare patients, the limitations related to staffing issues in many agencies limits this practice.

There are a significant number of patients being admitted for physical therapy, and these assessments include the discipline-specific information and address additional issues by virtue of OASIS. In a physical therapy evaluation conducted after a nursing admission, it may appear that there is almost a split personality at work. For example, the physical therapist may note issues with dyspnea and interfering pain that are often absent from an evaluation. Why would those same issues not be relevant regardless of their formal inclusion of the OASIS document? In light of the continued concerns raised by Medicare as to the medical necessity of skilled therapy services, such disconnects in documentation tools and content miss a significant opportunity to link what therapists "typically" do with larger measurements of home health quality.

## Home Health Compare

When looking at the Home Health Compare outcome scores, accessible to anyone at *www.medicare.gov,* it can be tempting to gravitate toward some more than others. Areas that are scored include the following:

- Improvement in ambulation
- Improvement in bed transfer
- Improvement in pain interfering with activity
- Improvement in bathing
- Improvement in management of oral medications
- Improvement in dyspnea
- Improvement in the status of surgical wounds
- Acute care hospitalizations
- Emergency department use without hospitalization

The outcome relating to ambulation appears to be physical therapy, bathing would be occupational therapy, and oral medication would be nursing. However, there is a flaw in this plan, as not every home health patient receives nursing and not every home health patient receives therapy. Based on utilization, it is not possible to hold one specific discipline responsible for one specific outcome. The team approach is key to effective care delivery, which creates solid documentation as an end product. OASIS items collect data elements, but they do not explain why a problem exists. That is left to clinical judgment, which then triggers which discipline or mix of disciplines is the most effective and efficient for each individual patient.

Since 2000, agencies have been challenged to embrace the idea of interfering pain. Healthcare providers are very familiar and comfortable with using the 0–10 pain scale in all settings. Patients are so used to this scale that they may even greet the therapist arriving at the home with "I am a 5 today" without even being asked. Level of pain is an important component of the assessment, but the outcome measure related to pain is not tied to or driven by a number. It is a noble goal to decrease a patient's pain level in every case, but that may not be realistic given the population serviced by home health.

### OASIS (M1242)

The Home Health Compare outcome is measured by the following OASIS item:
Frequency of pain interfering with patient's activity or movement:

- ❑ 0 – Patient has no pain
- ❑ 1 – Patient has pain that does not interfere with activity or movement
- ❑ 2 – Less often than daily
- ❑ 3 – Daily, but not constantly
- ❑ 4 – All of the time

As can be seen in the item, there is no mention of a pain level. Instead, the focus is on how the pain, regardless of level, is interfering with the patient's function and quality of life. It is possible that a patient would rate her pain as "0" because she is sitting still and has just taken her medications. Pressing further, a therapist might determine that pain is worse in the morning and makes dressing a much more difficult task. The score for M1242 would be response "3" despite a current pain level being reported as "0." As we work with this patient and provide occupational therapy to address the dressing issues, we can change how pain is affecting her life. At discharge, she reports much less difficulty with dressing, so her M1242 score would show improvement compared to the admission score.

During the discharge visit, she reports a pain level of "2," and the therapist may begin to panic. It appears that she is "worse" because her pain level went up, but the outcome being pursued is pain management in the functional and quality of life areas. A lower pain level at discharge is a good thing, but that is not the measurement of the outcome "improvement in pain." Here is the gap: Does a therapist only think along these lines when completing an OASIS but not on a therapy evaluation? The overwhelming majority of therapy evaluation tools collect information about level of pain, what makes it worse, what makes it better, and so on. What is missing is the link between pain and interference. With therapy being obviously tied to function, the impact of pain on these tasks should be evident in the documentation and consistent with the OASIS responses.

Along similar lines is the issue of dyspnea. OASIS data collection in this area is not directly tied to any specific pulmonary diagnosis. Think about a time when you have had a bad cold or flu and been in bed for several days. When you start to feel better, the stairs in your home can seem like a mountain, and climbing up them can result in shortness of breath. This experience does not necessarily indicate that you are acquiring a pulmonary disease; rather, it is a byproduct of inactivity due to illness. The OASIS item asks for the level of activity that provokes the shortness of breath.

**OASIS (M1400)**

When is the patient dyspneic or noticeably short of breath?

- ❑ 0 – Patient is not short of breath
- ❑ 1 – When walking more than 20 feet, climbing stairs
- ❑ 2 – With moderate exertion (e.g., while dressing, using commode or bedpan, walking distances less than 20 feet)
- ❑ 3 – With minimal exertion (e.g., while eating, talking, or performing other ADLs) or with agitation
- ❑ 4 – At rest (during day or night)

Agencies have spent a significant amount of time educating clinicians who complete admissions on this particular item, with the end result that many admissions report that the patient is a response 2 (with moderate exertion). Within days of the admission visit by nursing, the physical therapist completes an evaluation, which includes information that the patient is ambulating 50 feet with standby assistance and a walker but with no mention at all of shortness of breath. It is possible that the patient did not present with dyspnea on the therapy evaluation, but it is also possible that the therapist was not thinking about and ultimately documenting these findings as part of a complete assessment. For occupational therapy, awareness of dyspnea as a component of assessing dressing and other self-care tasks is a key element. Shortness of breath while speaking, if present, should show up as part of the speech-language pathology evaluation.

Therapists also must consider issues that the patient may have and that can complicate the plan of care. The cognitive behavioral section of OASIS has often been artificially connected to patient diagnosis. As an example, a patient diagnosed with dementia is more likely to have scores reflecting issues with memory or confusion, while the patient who does not have a diagnosis along those lines is scored as not having any issues. Consider the following OASIS item:

### OASIS (M1700)

**Cognitive Functioning:** Patient's current (day of assessment) level of alertness, orientation, comprehension, concentration, and immediate memory for simple commands.

- ❑ 0 – Alert/oriented, able to focus and shift attention, comprehends and recalls task directions independently.
- ❑ 1 – Requires prompting (cuing, repetition, reminders) only under stressful or unfamiliar conditions.
- ❑ 2 – Requires assistance and some direction in specific situations (e.g., on all tasks involving shifting of attention) or consistently requires low stimulus environment due to distractibility.
- ❑ 3 – Requires considerable assistance in routine situations. Is not alert and oriented or is unable to shift attention and recall directions more than half the time.
- ❑ 4 – Totally dependent due to disturbances such as constant disorientation, coma, persistent vegetative state, or delirium.

Notice that there is no mention of a diagnosis but rather a focus on the current level of alertness *and* orientation, comprehension, concentration, and immediate memory for simple commands. A review of records indicates that clinicians may only be reading as far as the first few words of response 0 ("alert and oriented") while not looking at the rest of that response, which addresses attention, comprehension, and recall. In reality, many patients are fine with information they already know, but teaching about wound care or a home program may be a different situation. The clinician needs to understand that by selecting response 0, Medicare is being told that the patient can also recall task directions independently. If that is true, consider how much repeat training the patient would actually require. Also consider how the medical necessity of repeat visits for teaching would be supported. This is not to say that no home health patients should be scored as "0," but clinicians need to recognize that if repeated teaching of new information will be required, a response of "1" would be more appropriate.

Moving to the therapy documentation specifically, issues of memory, attention, and recall are often absent unless there is a related diagnosis that ends up in the current or past medical history information. If the initial assessment includes this information, it would be reasonable to expect to see it impact the plan of care and the delivery of care on subsequent visits. The sheer number of questions related to cognitive behavioral issues in OASIS indicates that Medicare is looking for information reflecting the complexity of the patients being served, and this level of detail will provide additional support for skilled care.

Management of oral medications raises issues previously touched upon with respect to scope of practice, but it is imperative to fully understand the OASIS items and responses involved in determining improvement in this area.

## OASIS (M2020)

**Management of Oral Medications:** Patient's current ability to prepare and take all oral medications reliably and safely, including administration of the correct dosage at the appropriate times/intervals. Excludes injectable and IV medications. (Note: This refers to ability, not compliance or willingness.)

- ❑ 0 – Able to independently take the correct oral medication(s) and proper dosage(s) at the correct times.
- ❑ 1 – Able to take medication(s) at the correct times if:
  - ❑ (a) individual dosages are prepared in advance by another person; OR
  - ❑ (b) another person develops a drug diary or chart.
- ❑ 2 – Able to take medication(s) at the correct times if given reminders by another person at the appropriate times.
- ❑ 3 – Unable to take medication unless administered by another person.
- ❑ NA – No oral medications prescribed.

There is no mention in the item of the patient being able to recite his or her entire medication list by memory, including the chemical composition of each. Limited knowledge of the proper medication regimen may be a contributing factor impacting oral medication management, but one cannot overlook the functionality of this item. When assessing gait, has the physical therapist asked the patient where he or she keeps her medications? If they are in the bathroom upstairs and the patient has to take them three times per day, is he or she able to access them safely, or would assistance be necessary? Occupational therapy is closely tied to fine-motor skills, and these are clearly relevant to the act of opening pill bottles. Should the occupational therapy evaluation show routine assessment of this task, as it can have a significant impact on patient safety and hospitalization risks? The speech therapy evaluation may highlight issues with memory or problem solving, but how does that impact medication management? All three disciplines have the potential to make a positive impact on this specific outcome depending on "why" the issue exists, yet little information about medication management is clearly documented by any of them as part of the assessment or the plan of care.

Home health has been directed by Medicare to be an active participant in reducing rehospitalization rates, and that is reflected in the outcome measure specific to this issue. There is an OASIS item that should be considered as part of an agency's efforts to decrease this rate. It also represents the challenge of interdisciplinary care management.

**OASIS (M1033)**

**Risk for Hospitalization:** Which of the following signs or symptoms characterize the patient as at risk for hospitalization? (Mark all that apply.)

- ❑ 1 – History of falls (2 or more falls—or any fall with an injury—in the past 12 months
- ❑ 2 – Unintentional weight loss of a total of 10 pounds or more in the past 2 months
- ❑ 3 – Multiple hospitalizations (2 or more) in the past 6 months
- ❑ 4 – Multiple emergency department visits (2 or more) in the past 6 months
- ❑ 5 – Decline in mental, emotional, or behavioral status in the past 3 months
- ❑ 6 – Reported or observed history of difficulty complying with any medical instructions (for example, medications, diet, exercise) in the past 3 months
- ❑ 7 – Currently taking 5 or more medications
- ❑ 8 – Currently reports exhaustion
- ❑ 9 – Other risk(s) not listed in 1–8
- ❑ 10 – None of the above

This information is collected at the start of care by the admitting clinician. Once complete, it will be subject to the review process and then transmitted to Medicare. If an agency is truly working on decreasing preventable hospitalizations, having this information available only to the clinician who did the admission and to the review staff would not be the best use of this data. Capturing risks should translate into a plan of care to address them individually for each patient and to trigger the inclusion of other services to assist as indicated. Some will report challenges to accessing this information or say that they do not even know for sure who did the admission. This item and the follow-up it implies embody interdisciplinary patient-focused care and highlight the primary roadblocks many agencies and clinicians struggle with: communication, collaboration, and documentation.

## Connecting OASIS to Therapy

No one is suggesting that therapists in home health will love the OASIS and jump for joy at the opportunity to be involved in data collection. It is a unique tool that requires both baseline and ongoing training, but it must shift from being perceived as "extra" work to being perceived as an integral part of care delivery, with the patient at the center. The tool provides insight to therapy as to larger outcome measurement issues, which they are uniquely qualified to address. Being an active participant in collecting accurate data and showing consistency in discipline-specific documentation will better support the medical necessity and inclusion of therapy services in the plan of care designed to meet the needs of each individual patient.

 

Chapter 5

# Assessments: The Foundation for Medical Necessity

## Homebound Status

In order to qualify for home-based services to be paid for under the Medicare benefit, the patient has to be "homebound." Homebound status must be determined at the time of the admission assessment and periodically over the course of care. This task is not conducted exclusively by the discipline that completed the start of care visit; rather, it is the responsibility of all clinicians to confirm that the patient qualifies for services throughout the 60-day episode.

Being homebound does not mean confined to bed, nor does it imply that the patient is a home hostage. Discharge is not suddenly mandatory the minute the patient crosses the threshold and steps outside. The regulations themselves do not contain a list of approved places where the patient may go and acceptable durations of time for which the patient can be out of the home. Instead, there are three main components to homebound status that should be considered simultaneously, and none of them is tied to destination.

**1. Infrequent.** The patient who is considered homebound may nevertheless be away from the home periodically. However, if he or she is able to leave the home regularly for other activities, then he or she should be capable of accessing medical care—therapy, nursing, or social work—on an outpatient basis. When that is the case, he or she no longer qualifies for home services. The regulations do not specify any particular number of days, so frequency must be discussed with the patient over the course of care. When the interdisciplinary team confirms a regular pattern of time away from home, they should consider discharging the patient from home-based services.

**2. Short duration.** For a patient to be considered homebound, any time that he or she spends outside the home should be brief. It should not last for hours on end or occur routinely (see "infrequent"). Again, the home health benefit is designed for people who cannot access necessary medical care outside the home, so those who are able to spend significant amounts of time outside the home would not qualify. The regulations do not specify acceptable lengths of time, so clinicians must assess each individual patient and determine what his or her status may be in this area.

**3. Taxing effort.** The physical demands, psychosocial issues, and/or safety concerns of leaving the home are high enough that they limit the patient's ability to receive necessary medical care outside of the home. This component probably carries the greatest weight with respect to confirming homebound status. Here are some examples:

a. Mr. Anderson is unable to walk more than 30 feet with his walker before he becomes very short of breath and must sit to rest. His ability to participate effectively in outpatient therapy is insufficient at this time, as he fatigues quickly.

b. Mrs. Greyhound has pain in both of her hips and requires her daughter's assistance to dress and bathe. Her pain becomes intolerable when riding in a car for more than 10 minutes, and her home is more than 30 minutes away from her physician's office. She is new to Coumadin and requires regular lab draws as well as significant monitoring and education, but she cannot get to her doctor to meet these needs at this time.

c. Mr. Peterson has issues with anxiety, but when he keeps his regular routine, he is able to function fairly well without major incidents. He fell at home about a month ago and needs follow-up on lower extremity biomechanics, but the initial attempts at outpatient physical therapy were unsuccessful: They made him so upset that he could not participate.

To clarify the homebound issue, a patient cannot simply decide that he or she wants to stay home and receive care in a way that is more convenient. As illustrated in the examples provided, various issues can cause a person to be homebound. That is why the clinical decision-making skills of a nurse or therapist are required to determine the appropriate level of care for a patient.

Medicare has been asked to provide further clarity on the homebound issue, and the end result has been a list of examples. "Examples" is the key word, as they do not serve as a checklist of "approved" locations or activities. The patient is allowed to leave the home for medically related appointments, to attend church services, to get their hair done, to go for a walk around the block, or to participate in family events such as birthdays, weddings, holidays, and funerals. Keep in mind that homebound status is not tied to any specific destination and must be confirmed based on frequency of leaving the home, duration of absences, and the amount of effort it takes to complete the activity.

Here are some examples to consider:

1. Mrs. Matthews is a Medicare recipient and has orders for home health. This past week, she went to get her hair done and stopped to visit with her friend for her recent birthday. She went to church and had her routine physician appointment as well. She completed all of these tasks with few problems, and as she has not driven in the past five years, her daughter drove her to all of these locations. Despite the fact that all of those activities appear on the example list from Medicare, Mrs. Matthews would not meet the homebound criteria. She is leaving the home regularly, she is gone for varying amounts of time, and leaving does not require significant effort.

2. Mr. Patten is a Medicare recipient and has orders for home health. Yesterday, he went to the grocery store with his son. He does so once or twice a month, as it involves picking up his medications and he likes to talk about them with the pharmacist. On this recent trip, he was able to walk into the store, but he became very fatigued. The son secured one of the scooters from the store, but Mr. Patten was unable to maneuver it safety due to pain in his hands and some newly emerging cognitive issues. He ended up waiting in the car while his son bought the necessary items. Once home, Mr. Patten went to take a nap and later complained of increased pain in both hands and his legs, which is still present today, despite his having taken his pain medications correctly. Mr. Patten would be considered homebound even though grocery shopping is not mentioned on the Medicare list of examples. He leaves home infrequently, and doing so clearly takes taxing effort. It is unrealistic for him to access medical care on an outpatient basis at this time to address his needs.

The determination and confirmation of homebound status is a key component of assessments and of routine visits for all three therapy disciplines. As an integral part of the documentation, carefully consider what makes leaving the home a "taxing effort." It is also important to keep homebound status in its proper place: It is a key aspect of the Medicare coverage criteria, but it is not the goal of home health providers to keep patients at that level.

It can be difficult for providers to remember the ultimate goal, however, when patients fear that they will lose care they've come to rely on. Think about how a patient is introduced to the concept of homebound status: It occurs on the admission visit, which many will report is routinely an hour and a half to two hours. Amid all of the questions being asked, papers being signed, and tasks being demonstrated, the patient is basically read the Miranda rights of home health—that is, if the patient gets better and can leave the home, the agency will discharge. This message is delivered at the very first interaction with the patient and plants the idea that progress is not necessarily a good thing. Patients are probably at their sickest when services begin and are told that recovery will mean loss of services. For some patients, this is not a problem, as they are more than motivated to discontinue services as soon as they are able. Others appreciate the care so much that they do not want it to end for quite some time. Home health therapists can get caught up in this idea and miss the true purpose of providing skilled care, which is to improve the patient's situation so that they are no longer homebound.

There have been questions raised about the level of ability that a person must have to function in the community. The following list of questions is based on an article entitled "Defining Community Ambulation From the Perspective of the Older Adult" *(Journal of Geriatric PT* 33(2):56–63, April/June 2010). The intention of this list is to help therapists plan care for home health patients and consider how they may want to function after discharge from services:

Can the patient:

- ❑ Carry a 5-pound weight for >1,000 feet?
- ❑ Carry packages averaging 6–7 pounds for short distances?
- ❑ Walk a minimum of 1,000 feet per errand for two to three errands per trip?
- ❑ Change speeds and maintain balance?
- ❑ Negotiate safely around obstacles, slopes, or curbs while looking in a variety of directions?
- ❑ Multitask while walking (walk and talk, walk and look from side to side or up and down)?
- ❑ Carry a package up and down the stairs?
- ❑ Safely engage in postural transitions, such as changing directions, reaching, looking up or down or sideways, or moving backwards?
- ❑ Rise from a chair without the use of arms with minimal effort?

 

- ❑ Walk at 4 feet per second for at least one minute to cross a street?
- ❑ Walk at a minimum speed of 160 feet per minute or about 2.6 feet per second?

When looking over this list, there is at least one item that can make even the most seasoned home health therapist pause: the ability to walk distances of 1,000 feet. It is critical to put this issue in the most functional perspective possible. Consider how much a therapist walks on any given day. How far is it from where your parked the car to the office? Or from your car into the grocery store? There are no distance limitations in the homebound definition, so clinicians must consider each unique patient situation to determine whether the patient is fully able to participate effectively in medical care outside the home.

## Initiating the Assessment

Routinely seen as problem solvers, therapists can provide interventions without even thinking about it, and when documentation occurs after that point, the assessment may no longer be accurate or clearly in support of the need for skilled care. For example, while assessing Mr. Jasper's ability to get on and off the toilet, the therapist sees that he is struggling to complete the task safely. The toilet is much too low for him, and he is trying to push himself up with the toilet paper hanger and the vanity. Noticing the bedside commode in the dining room, the therapist asks Mr. Jasper whether it is okay to show him how to use the frame over the toilet. He agrees. Once it is in place, he attempts the transfer again and is now able to complete the task safely and independently. Later that day, the therapist is completing the assessment note. For toilet transfers, the therapist documents Mr. Jasper's ability as "independent with a commode frame in place." But is this correct? Before a skilled intervention was provided, the therapist noted safety concerns and the need for assistance—and that is what should have been documented. The instruction and relocation of the commode frame would still be documented but in a different area of the visit. If the level of ability is, in fact, documented as independent, then the intervention and skill of the therapist specific to that task is lost. Timing of documentation completion as well as clarity about what defines the patient's true ability can enhance or detract from medical necessity.

### *Prior level of function*

Regardless of who completes the assessment—the physical therapist, occupational therapist, or speech-language pathologist—one element that must always be documented is the patient's prior level of function (PLOF). Agencies are reporting that when attempts are made to appeal a denial for payment of therapy services rendered, PLOF is being looked at closely, especially at the Administrative Law Judge (ALJ) level. Absence of this information does not strengthen the case for skilled therapy; instead, it raises concerns about how much improvement could realistically be expected when a baseline level with time frames is not documented.

Therapists typically cite one of two reasons for not documenting PLOF. The first is that they were not present to confirm what the patient and/or caregiver reports, so they are unsure whether it is accurate. The second is a concern that if their interventions improve a patient beyond the documented PLOF, then they will be at risk for payment denial. As to the accuracy of self-reported information, this is a risk for both prior and current functional abilities, but that does not reduce its importance. It is understood that the details are not based on the therapist's direct observation, and if there are questions as to accuracy, the therapist can document that fact. Regarding the second issue, it is entirely possible that the interventions can help the patient attain a higher than expected level of functional ability, especially if there were few or no interventions for a considerable length of time. Once again, this does not make documentation of PLOF optional, as goals can be updated and should be supported in the medical record to indicate why skilled care would continue to be effective. PLOF provides a general context for performance and a baseline expectation to support the necessity of therapy interventions.

Compare these two patients:

1. Mr. Adams is 70 years old and fell out of bed, fracturing his left hip. He was taken to the emergency room and admitted later that day for a hip pinning. Prior to this fall, he was taking daily walks with no assistive device around the assisted living facility in which he resides, and he routinely participated in community outings. Currently, he can only walk about 5 feet with his walker, has considerable pain, and has substantial issues with maintaining his weight-bearing restriction. The physical therapy gait goal is 300 feet with a cane independently.

2. Mr. Addams is 70 years old and fell out of bed, fracturing his left hip. He was taken to the emergency room and admitted later that day for a hip pinning. Prior to this fall, he required minimal assistance to transfer from his bed to a scooter, which was his primary method of mobility for the past five years due to severe arthritis. Other than taking a few steps as part of the transfer process, he has not been a functional ambulator. He currently requires moderate assistance to

 

complete transfers safely. The physical therapy gait goal is 300 feet with a cane independently.

The patients' ages, injuries, and surgical follow-ups are intentionally the same. PLOF clearly created two different expectations as to what level of activity could reasonably be expected for each patient. Although the goals for physical therapy are identical, the first appears appropriate, while the second does not.

### *Prior level of care*

There is another "prior level" that needs to be considered when completing assessments—the prior level of care. When a patient has been in a rehabilitation unit, skilled nursing facility, or other setting while receiving therapy services and is then referred to home health for therapy services, it is expected that a certain amount of skilled care has already been provided. As such, there needs to be a clear reason to support continued therapy services. Although there is no limitation on the number of visits in this situation, the payer source has already been billed for therapy care, so clear support is necessary to justify continued services.

The single biggest difference between a patient's level of function within a facility setting and his or her level of function within the home is not a sudden onset of "weakness," but rather the unique challenges presented by the home environment. Assisting a patient in the transitional process—applying what they learned within a facility to real-world situations—can be the primary focus of home health, as well as building upon the prior level of care to reach new heights. These challenges may include structural, psychosocial, and economic concerns, as well as the general distractions of daily life (e.g., dealing with pets, grandchildren, having the television on). Understanding these challenges is essential in explaining why a therapist is needed to facilitate a positive and safe transition.

Switching gears, consider the patient who has not received therapy services prior to his or her home health referral. In this case, the expected plan is to start from scratch, which may present additional issues that therapy must address, as there has been no formal intervention to this point. Note that this does not necessarily mean that such a patient will require more visits than a patient who received therapy prior to home health admission. The therapist is still compelled to make the case for skilled care, but the expectations are different.

The following table pulls together both "prior level" concepts. Taking all perceived payer expectations and any regulations out of the discussion, any therapist completing an assessment must consider both of these concepts, as both are relevant and should ultimately be part of the documentation.

FIGURE 5.1 **Impact of Prior Level**

| Prior level of function | Prior level of care |
|---|---|
| • Creates context | • Creates expectations |
| • Time frame is significant | • Time spent is significant |
| • Mostly self-reported | • Self-report and notes |
| • Is NOT the cutoff for rehab potential | • Does NOT define rehab potential |

### *Use of 'independent'*

One specific term has contributed to confusion regarding the need for therapy services: "independent." At first glance, it can be hard to see why this word would be an issue, as it appears to be straightforward: It simply means the patient is able to complete a given task consistently, without assistance of any kind and without safety concerns, whenever he or she chooses to do it. Being independent implies that there is no need for skilled intervention in a particular area. Although therapists may believe that this term is being used correctly in assessment documentation, consider these examples from real records:

- "Independent but unsafe"
- "Independent but unsteady"
- "Independent with supervision"
- "Independent but requires repeated attempts"
- "Independent with verbal cues"

There is no place in therapy documentation for "independent but ..." or for combining independent with other levels of assistance, such as supervision and verbal cues. A patient is either independent or not—there is no halfway.

 

### *Subjective information*

Much like PLOF, subjective information is integral to a thorough therapy assessment. In numerous record reviews, however, it appears that the amount of subjective information being collected is declining, and in some cases, such information is completely absent.

As healthcare reform continues to reinforce the concept of patient-focused care, therapists need to pay attention to what patients have to say about their prior and current level of ability, how they feel about their situation, and what they hope to achieve by participating in therapy. Patients can, on occasion, talk for quite a long time about topics such as their bowels, and it can be a challenge to help them focus on a particular question. Nevertheless, their participation in a therapy assessment is more than physical demonstration. Compliance with the ultimate plan of care is enhanced when the patient is part of the process and when his or her goals are recognized and included.

## Comprehensive Assessments

Those who complete assessments in the home setting are responsible for managing the whole patient, not just one aspect of his or her well-being. For therapists, this responsibility raises questions about what areas fall within their scope of practice and what should be included in the documentation, beyond the traditional elements of strength, mobility, and self-management. Before taking on those "therapy" areas in more detail, there are basic pieces of patient information that any of the therapies practicing in home health should consider as part of routine assessments.

### *Medical history*

Recording the patient's medical history creates a picture of the individual's overall health status and identifies factors that may impact the course of care. Including the diagnosis codes that are used for the home health episode shows consistency with the overall plan of care.

### *Vital signs*

Vital signs include blood pressure, pulse, and respirations. For patients identified with or prone to infections, consider taking temperature readings as well. Patient-specific parameters and criteria for physician notification should be documented and communicated to all clinicians involved with the plan of care. These pieces of information provide insight into the general health of the patient and can be indicators of emerging issues. Given the amount of activity that can occur during a therapy evaluation, readings before and after activity as well as before and after position change can provide important details about the patient's status and reaction to treatment. Therapists need to be trained on how to take vital signs correctly and consistently, demonstrate competence, and be provided with the appropriate equipment to complete these tasks.

### *Pain*

Sometimes referred to as the "fifth vital sign," assessment of pain extends beyond collecting data using the 0–10 pain scale. Many patients are so accustomed to being asked to provide a number in a variety of healthcare settings that they will volunteer "I am a 5" without even having to be asked, but that information is not enough. Nearly every therapy evaluation form includes current level of pain, what impacts it, and what the patient is doing to manage it, and that information is important, even though those these questions are often left blank. Connecting back to OASIS, it's also helpful to determine how pain affects the patient's ability to function. Has any activity or task been done less often or stopped completely in an attempt to manage pain? This information can be specifically relevant to physical therapy, occupational therapy, and speech-language pathology and increases the connections between traditional therapy assessments and meaningful patient information.

### *Medications*

The therapist should review the medication profile to determine whether there are any potential issues that could impact the therapy plan of care. With some medications, for example, side effects include fatigue and weakness, and neither may be corrected with only a routine exercise program. Also consider the functionality that patients require in order to take medications properly—ambulation skills to access them, fine-motor skills to handle them, and cognitive skills to remember when and how to take them. Document according to agency policy any changes in the regimen with respect to dosing, frequency, or addition/removal of a medication.

### *Wounds*

Including information about the presence of a wound or wounds does not necessarily imply that active wound care is part of the therapy plan. Nevertheless, that information is important because the location and status of a wound could directly affect the patient's ability to tolerate therapy activities. Certain precautions, such as not getting the area wet, could impact self-care. They may also provide information: The existence of pressure ulcers may indicate a need to improve mobility to promote healing. If a risk for pressure ulcers has been identified, then the need to minimize or eliminate the contributing factors increases the support for addressing these issues through skilled therapy services.

### *Incontinence*

The presence of incontinence may indicate physiological issues, but the underlying cause may be related to mobility and self-care. A patient who is new to using a walker may find gait velocity decreased, or he or she may find that the walker does not fit easily through doorways, and these delays can trigger bladder "accidents" that were not an issue in the past. New onset of fatigue or weakness can contribute to challenges with toileting hygiene and increase fall risk when performing these tasks. Cognitive and communication issues can disrupt a timed voiding program or make it more difficult to know when the patient needs to be taken to the bathroom. These are very real and functional issues for patients, and depending on the findings of the assessment, each therapy discipline can bring a set of skills to the table.

## Connecting the Dots

A traditional therapy assessment covers all of the basic areas of measurement, such as strength, balance, range of motion, and cognition, by providing a separate and distinct area for each. Other areas of the form, whether electronic or on paper, will contain sections for functional activities such as ambulation, dressing, bathing, swallowing, and memory. There is an assumption that the reader of the assessment will know which deficits connect to which functional problem. The question is: How well does that actually work in terms of communicating each therapy discipline's unique skill set? The therapist must  do a more thorough job of connecting the dots.

Consider these examples:

- Patient A requires moderate assistance to shower safely. He has macular degeneration that makes it difficult to see the temperature controls clearly. He also has a balance issue that causes him to rely heavily on the shower wall to steady himself.

- Patient B requires moderate assistance to shower safely. He fell in the shower a week ago and is very anxious about being in that situation again. He is in need of a transfer bench.
- Patient C requires moderate assistance to shower safely. He had rotator cuff surgery recently and is unable to use his left arm actively at this time. He has significant pain issues and complains of some dizziness after taking his medications.

In all three situations, the patient requires moderate assistance to shower safely. However, the reasons for this level of assistance vary greatly, as would the plans for addressing them. The problem is that many current therapy evaluations stop at designating the level of assistance and do not connect it to the measurable components that are causing the problems with a functional task. This approach contributes to assessments that contain limited skilled detail and that appear repetitive upon review. It takes the skills and experience of a therapist to see beyond the single piece of information (e.g., the level of assistance) to the underlying cause. These details make the assessment distinctly therapy and show that the care specific to each individual patient is indispensable.

## Objective Measurements

The 2011 Home Health PPS Final Rule reinforces that therapists are expected to be as objective as possible when collecting assessment information. Range of motion and strength assessments are great examples of tools that can be considered objective in some situations and not in others. The methods that therapists are taught for collecting range of motion (using the goniometer and bony landmarks) and strength (manual muscle testing using the 0–5 scale) are objective. However, if the therapist chooses to use percentages, writes general comments, or fails to be specific, then the information is no longer objective.

In any discussion of formal testing, understanding some key terminology is required. "Standardized" indicates that the assessment is completed in a defined way and that it is used every time the data are collected. Examples include manual muscle testing and range of motion assessments. "Validated" tools have research behind them to support that the scoring or findings mean something real and are not random data. Look into the available research to determine for which patient population, such as community-dwelling elderly, a given tool is validated and to confirm that it's relevant for a given patient. Clarity around "standardized" and "validated" has been a challenge in home health, specifically in relation to fall risk assessments.

Tests and measures for therapy are not required to be both standardized and validated, nor are specific purchased tools required. Selection of tools is at the discretion of the therapist completing the assessment, and he or she should take care to select tools that provide meaningful information and that are actively used in care planning, rather than simply completing them to meet a requirement. In addition, when a test or measurement is completed at the time of the initial assessment, it should be repeated at a point later in the episode and at least at the time of discharge to confirm the impact of care.

**Remember:** Reporting a test score or listing a strength grade is not enough. There needs to be an *analysis* of that data, along with a clear connection of these findings to the care plan, which supports why therapy is necessary.

## Therapy-Specific Assessments

Moving into the therapy-specific assessment areas will impact each of the three therapies differently. When more than one therapy is providing care, the different disciplines may focus their attention differently, but it is imperative that the message being conveyed about the patient be consistent. Inconsistency sows the seeds of doubt about the assessment's accuracy and can lead to payment denials. For example, the occupational therapist documents that the patient is ambulating "ad lib" in the home with no equipment or safety concerns. Meanwhile, the physical therapist documents a plan for eight visits to address fall risk and the need for gait training with a cane. The payer source will likely lean toward the occupational therapist's assessment and deny the need for physical therapy. It's not essential for all three therapy assessments to contain identical information, but when other services are required, each assessment should support inclusion of those services. This is a fundamental component of supporting the need for skilled intervention as a team.

The following are several key areas specific to physical therapy, occupational therapy, and speech-language pathology assessments. This list is not all inclusive, as there can and should be variation in specific patient populations, but it is meant to facilitate improved transition from clinical decision-making to documentation to support medical necessity.

# Physical Therapy

## *Gait*

Skilled gait assessments include the quality of the performance and not just the distance and device used. Assessment of stride length, weight shift, cadence, pelvic tilt, and balance are all examples of quality-related topics. Distance alone does not indicate that there is a deficit that must be addressed. For example, although 30 feet appears to be limited, the assessment must support the reason for the limitation and explain why physical therapy is needed to correct this issue. Having a patient walk a longer distance does not automatically require the skills of physical therapy—a caregiver might be able to do that. Similarly, 30 feet could be an adequate distance in a one-room dwelling, but it may not be adequate if the patient resides in an assisted living environment. Still, distance is a helpful metric: Some physical therapists omit distances completely from gait assessments, but when distance is removed, there is no measurable frame of reference and limited functional context for ambulation. A skilled gait assessment is a balance of both the quality and quantity of ambulation.

## *Transfers*

There are a variety of possible transfers within this assessment. The specific type of transfer, any relevant environmental components, level of assistance required, contributing factors, and the steps involved combine to reflect the skills of the therapist. Below is an outline of the key aspects of each transfer (this is not an exhaustive list). The assessment would contain the transfers relevant to the specific patient situation.

### Sit-to-stand transfer (recliner or kitchen chair)

- ❑ Surface height
- ❑ Use of support surfaces such as armrests
- ❑ Position of feet
- ❑ Ability to scoot forward
- ❑ Ability to shift weight
- ❑ Need for assistance (including "why")
- ❑ Number of attempts
- ❑ Fluidity of movement
- ❑ Ability to return to sitting position
- ❑ Safety throughout the task

 

### Tub/shower transfer

- ❑ Ability to position self for the transfer
- ❑ Use of/need for equipment
- ❑ If done from a seated position, include components of sit-to-stand transfer
- ❑ Need for assistance (including "why")
- ❑ Fluidity of movement
- ❑ Ability to exit the tub/shower
- ❑ Safety throughout the task

### Toilet transfer

- ❑ Surface height
- ❑ Use of support surfaces such as grab bars or counters
- ❑ Ability to position self in front of toilet
- ❑ Ability to sit down smoothly and safely
- ❑ Need for assistance (including "why")
- ❑ Number of attempts
- ❑ Fluidity of movement
- ❑ Ability to return to standing position
- ❑ Safety throughout the task

### Bed to chair transfer

- ❑ Ability to move from supine to a sitting position, including level of assist and why assist is needed
- ❑ Ability to stabilize self in seated position at edge of bed
- ❑ Ability to shift weight properly
- ❑ Use of/need for equipment
- ❑ Need for assistance (including "why")
- ❑ Ability to position self in front of next seating surface
- ❑ Ability to return to sitting, including level of assist and why assist is needed
- ❑ Safety throughout the task

**Other transfers to consider:**

- ❑ Car transfers—key to ability to access medical care outside the home
- ❑ Getting up from the floor—important aspect of fall recovery training
- ❑ Wheelchair transfers—use of a wheelchair as part of transfers will change some of the components and should be documented with that level of detail

### *Bed mobility*

Assessment of bed mobility is often documented by level of assistance only. Ability to turn and position self in bed involves the components of rolling, bridging, and scooting. The "why" behind the level of assist may vary between components and should be documented when this is a problem area for a patient.

### *Fall risk*

The risk for falls is based on multiple factors and is not confirmed by gait distances or a general scoring of balance (e.g., F-). Each patient has a unique set of risk factors, and those factors should drive the selection of interventions to decrease risks in a meaningful way. Factors include but are not limited to the following:

- ❑ Medication regimen
- ❑ Environmental issues
- ❑ Weakness
- ❑ Balance deficits
- ❑ Visual issues
- ❑ Cognitive issues
- ❑ History and context of previous falls
- ❑ Dizziness/vertigo

### *Self-care*

Although some professionals may assert that occupational therapy addresses self-care areas more specifically, documenting these areas as "deferred to OT" or omitting them completely misses an opportunity to connect deficit areas with functional issues. In addition, including this area supports the need for a referral to occupational therapy with objective data. Pay attention to why assistance is needed in areas such as dressing, bathing, meal prep, and medication management.

 

### Balance

Formal tests are used more often in this area of the physical therapy assessment and include but are not limited to the Tinetti, the Berg Balance Assessment, the Timed Up and Go, and the 6-Minute Walk Test. These serve a much clearer purpose than do general comments such as "good," "fair," and "poor." Physical therapists must follow these standardized tools and cannot modify them on their own. It is important that physical therapists be competent and comfortable with any tool selected, keeping in mind that they may choose from a variety of tools.

### Strength

Current documentation of manual muscle testing at times appears to be more of a screening than a true muscle-by-muscle formal assessment. This fact does not make a screening inappropriate, but the therapist should be clear that testing muscle groups is not the same as conducting isolated testing. The screening model should be a trigger for a more detailed assessment as indicated. "Muscle weakness" is not an observation; it must have measurable data behind it as well as a clear connection to the impact on a meaningful functional activity.

### Muscle tone

Although deemed to not be an issue for many home health patients, muscle tone may actually be more of an issue than it seems. Inactivity can lead to atrophy over time, and in the growing population of patients who are of advanced age entering home health, one wonders whether this component of a physical therapy assessment is being utilized correctly.

### Range of motion

Documentation of active and passive range of motion requires goniometry, utilizing specified landmarks for any joint being assessed. This method meets the expectation of a standardized assessment. Note, however, that both too little and too much detail are both problematic: Estimating, eyeballing, or labeling "with functional limitations" or "WFL" does not meet the expectation, but when the physical therapist regularly takes measurements to the level of the toe joints as part of the assessment, questions as to relevance and accuracy arise. For those reasons, the focus should be on problem areas as indicated and how they impact function.

 

### Endurance

Endurance has become a dirty word in therapy circles based on the belief that its use will trigger a payment denial. The issue is not the term itself, but rather in the fact that it has far too often been used in documentation. A classic example is an initial assessment that reads "Endurance: Fair" with a goal of "Endurance will be good." Moving from fair to good sounds like a measurable improvement, but key details are missing: What is that limited endurance keeping the patient from doing, and what will additional endurance mean for the patient's quality of life?

Instead of addressing the core issue, many therapists simply avoid the word "endurance" and replace it with "activity tolerance." The situation has not improved in any real way when assessments now read "Activity tolerance: Fair" with a goal of "Activity tolerance will be good." The core issue is the lack of clear connection to meaningful information from the patient's perspective. OASIS item M1400 reflects this issue in the area of dyspnea, as the item asks for the level of activity that provokes shortness of breath not tied to any specific pulmonary diagnosis. Therapy assessments should look at the dyspnea component of activity as well.

### Edema

Circumferential measurements with consistent landmarks and specific descriptors such as pitting, combined with any impact on mobility, create a skilled assessment of edema beyond a "mild" or "moderate" designation.

### Cognitive/behavioral

Issues with memory, alertness, depression, anxiety, and wandering are all relevant to successful execution of a physical therapy plan of care. Far too often, the information stops at the level of "alert and oriented" but may miss the opportunity to fully describe the complexities of the home health patient. The diagnosis label is not an actual assessment, and although focused interventions may not be part of the plan, more detail is needed. For example, a patient with depression may be feeling overwhelmed. The physical therapist may not be able to push this patient aggressively with respect to exercises and may need to keep the visits shorter to increase patient buy-in. The end result would be shorter visits than those for other patients and possibly more total visits in order to effectively manage this patient. Given the current environment in which providing more therapy visits is questioned as being driven by reimbursement, physical therapists must be clear in how cognitive and/or behavioral issues affect the plan of care.

 

### *Communication/comprehension*

A patient's ability to hear and understand communication as well as respond appropriately is a critical component of effective teaching strategies and is often overlooked in physical therapy assessment documentation. It appears that ownership of teaching as a key element of therapy interventions is not being documented consistently. Acknowledging any factors that could impede such communication or that will call for adjustments in delivery, such as less verbal and more written communication or the need to use pictures as opposed to words, demonstrates the set of skills necessary to manage the home health patient.

### *Environment*

The home health physical therapist understands the impact of the patient's environment on his or her ability to function. For example, the ability to ambulate in a facility's unobstructed, well-lit, linoleum-covered hallways does not automatically translate to the home, where clutter, throw rugs, and pets can create a whole new dynamic. Oxygen tubing can create exciting challenges to the task of maneuvering a walker, especially when the patient's beloved cat finds the dangling tube very interesting. These factors are very real issues for the patient, and when such relevant information is well documented, it supports the need for a skilled therapist to be involved with the plan of care.

### *Safety*

OASIS emphasizes the patient's safety when he or she is performing functional tasks. The challenge is to define safety in a way that is meaningful and specific to the patient. Simply calling a task "safe" or "unsafe" is not sufficient; the factors that make that task safe or unsafe must be included to reflect the skills of the therapist. Think about it this way: What is "safe" ambulation? For one patient, safety is maintained by using a walker and having two people assist. For another, it is the proper use of a cane when walking outdoors. For a third, proper footwear is key, as walking in slippers makes him unsteady and puts him at risk for falls. The prevalence of fall prevention programs and the referrals specific to physical therapy to address very real risks should be a launching point for the level of detail required. The term "safe" does not stand alone as a measurement.

### *Vision*

Much like cognition and communication, visual issues can directly affect both functional ability and teaching strategies. Visual issues are not limited to more obvious challenges, such as blindness. Consider how light sensitivity or macular degeneration in the diabetic patient can impact gait outdoors. The home program materials may need to be modified in order to be effective. Although vision may not be a specific physical therapy treatment area, it adds to the description of the unique and complex issues facing home health patients.

### Sensation

Evaluation of sensation was taught as a basic component of physical therapy assessments starting back in school, but many records include "intact" or "impaired" as the only response, with no additional information. Screening for such issues is important, however. A patient may not recognize the loss of sensation that has been gradually increasing over time. In addition, loss of proprioception can contribute significantly to gait issues and fall risk. The prevalence of diabetes reported for the home health population raises questions of underreporting of neuropathy issues by physical therapy, as it is unclear whether therapists routinely assess for such issues. OASIS-C added the process measure related to management of diabetic feet, which highlights Medicare's interest in how this issue is being handled in the home setting. Physical therapy should be an active participant in this area, as sensation assessments are key elements of being part of the interdisciplinary team.

## Occupational Therapy

### Activities of daily living (ADL)

It is vital that occupational therapists speak to individual self-care tasks and do not make generalized statements such as "min assist with ADLs." This practice misses the opportunity to demonstrate the potential variability in how specific patients perform tasks. In all of these activities, a complete assessment requires more than the level of assistance and must include "why" there is an issue. ADLs include but are not limited to the following:

- ❑ **Grooming:** Attention to cognitive and mobility components that can affect ability to groom safely.
- ❑ **Dressing:** As with OASIS, consider the ability to gather clothing items. Be aware of clothing choices to determine whether the items are what the patient routinely wears or reflect a modification based on difficulties encountered.
- ❑ **Bathing:** This task contains several components, so highlight the ones that are an issue, such as reaching a specific region of the body. Do not overlook any complicating factors, such as equipment needs, environmental concerns, or patient anxiety about bathing.

 

- **Toileting hygiene:** OASIS-C added a specific question about the ability to manage this important area of self-care, yet many occupational therapy documentation tools do not contain a distinct area for this information. Fall risk can increase when there are limited abilities in this set of tasks, thus increasing the need for therapy interventions.
- **Medication management:** As mentioned in the OASIS chapter, medication management is not exclusively about knowledge of side effects and timing of doses. Cognitive issues that impact these areas can and should be addressed by occupational therapy. When assessing fine-motor skills, routinely include specifics in relation to opening medication bottles or handling syringes to enhance the overall functional relevance of therapy interventions.
- **Feeding:** Assessment of self-feeding skills is not limited to neurologically impaired patients. Weakness or sensory issues in the upper extremities or sitting balance deficits can affect this area significantly.

### *Instrumental activities of daily living (IADL)*

Like ADLs, specificity and relevance are key components of a thorough occupational therapy assessment. In all of these activities, a complete assessment requires more than the level of assistance and must include "why" there is an issue. IADLs include but are not limited to the following:

- **Meal preparation:** There are many components of this task, so there are multiple opportunities for issues to arise. Food doesn't miraculously emerge from the refrigerator completely prepared. Gathering, carrying, preparing, and transporting food items can directly connect to fall risk and should be addressed as specific components.
- **Money management:** This area can be related to a patient's sense of self-worth and is clearly meaningful in some cases. Assessment can reflect cognitive and communication issues as well.
- **Household management:** Doing laundry, cleaning house, and managing home repair needs often appear to be dependent activities for home health patients based on the content of documentation. In the assessment documentation, distinguish between patient or caregiver report of performance and actual demonstration. Without such detail, it may appear that all of these tasks were attempted over the course of a single visit, which would be unrealistic in nearly all cases.

## Functional mobility

There has been a periodic debate between physical and occupational therapists about whether to include gait-related information in an occupational therapy assessment. Although physical therapy takes the lead on a detailed gait assessment, patients do walk during the course of many ADLs and IADLs, and lack of mobility information can make an occupational therapy assessment look incomplete. Take precautions to avoid generalized statements that may negatively impact the medical necessity of physical therapy, such as "patient ambulates ad lib," "patient ambulates independently," or "patient is independent with his cane," unless these statements are 100% accurate based on the definition of "independent" previously discussed. Challenges and concerns with mobility noted during ADLs should be noted and coordinated with other disciplines.

### *Transfers*

There are a variety of possible transfers within this assessment area. The specific type of transfer, any relevant environmental components, level of assistance required, contributing factors, and the steps involved combine to reflect the skills of the therapist. Below is an outline of the key aspects of each transfer (this is not an exhaustive list). The assessment would contain the transfers relevant to the specific patient situation.

#### *Sit-to-stand transfer (recliner or kitchen chair)*

- ❑ Surface height
- ❑ Use of support surfaces such as armrests
- ❑ Position of feet
- ❑ Ability to scoot forward
- ❑ Ability to shift weight
- ❑ Need for assistance (including "why")
- ❑ Number of attempts
- ❑ Fluidity of movement
- ❑ Ability to return to sitting position
- ❑ Safety throughout the task

#### *Tub/shower transfer*

- ❑ Ability to position self for the transfer
- ❑ Use of/need for equipment

 

- ❑ If done from seated position, include components of sit-to-stand transfer
- ❑ Need for assistance (including "why")
- ❑ Fluidity of movement
- ❑ Ability to exit the tub/shower
- ❑ Safety throughout the task

*Toilet transfer*

- ❑ Surface height
- ❑ Use of support surfaces such as grab bars or counters
- ❑ Ability to position self in front of toilet
- ❑ Ability to sit down smoothly and safely
- ❑ Need for assistance (including "why")
- ❑ Number of attempts
- ❑ Fluidity of movement
- ❑ Ability to return to standing position
- ❑ Safety throughout the task

*Bed to chair transfer*

- ❑ Ability to move from supine to a sitting position, including level of assist and why assist is needed
- ❑ Ability to stabilize self in seated position at edge of bed
- ❑ Ability to shift weight properly
- ❑ Use of/need for equipment
- ❑ Need for assistance (including "why")
- ❑ Ability to position self in front of next seating surface
- ❑ Ability to return to sitting, including level of assist and why assist is needed
- ❑ Safety throughout the task

### Other transfers to consider:

- ❑ Car transfers—key to ability to access medical care outside the home
- ❑ Getting up from the floor—important aspect of fall recovery training
- ❑ Wheelchair transfers—use of a wheelchair as part of transfers will change some of the components and should be documented with that level of detail

### Bed mobility

Assessment of bed mobility is often documented by level of assistance only. Ability to turn and position self in bed involves the components of rolling, bridging, and scooting. The "why" behind the level of assist may vary between components and should be documented when this is a problem area for a patient.

### Fall risk

The risk for falls is based on multiple factors and is not confirmed by gait distances or a general scoring of balance (e.g., F-). Each patient has a unique set of risk factors, and these factors should drive the selection of interventions to decrease risks in a meaningful way. Factors include but are not limited to the following:

- ❑ Medication regimen
- ❑ Environmental issues
- ❑ Weakness
- ❑ Balance deficits
- ❑ Visual issues
- ❑ Cognitive issues
- ❑ History and context of previous falls
- ❑ Dizziness/vertigo

#### Balance

Issues with balance in sitting and standing can significantly affect a variety of self-care tasks. Exercise caution when using the terms "poor," "fair," and "good" in relation to meaningful activity. For example, how would a patient with "poor" sitting balance be able to toilet independently? When collecting this information, keep in mind the larger picture of function.

#### Strength

When documenting strength, occupational therapists face a risk similar to the one that physical therapists face. Current documentation of manual muscle testing at times appears to be more of a screening than a true muscle-by-muscle formal assessment. This fact does not make a screening inappropriate, but the therapist should be clear that testing muscle groups is not the same as conducted isolated testing. The screening model should be a trigger for a more detailed assessment, as indicated. "Muscle weakness" is not an observation; it must have measurable data behind it as well as a clear connection to the impact on a meaningful self-care or household management activity.

### Muscle tone

Although deemed to not be an issue for many home health patients, muscle tone may actually be more of an issue than it seems. Inactivity can lead to atrophy over time, and in the growing population of patients who are of advanced age entering home health, one wonders whether this component of an occupational therapy assessment is being utilized correctly.

### Range of motion

Documentation of active and passive range of motion requires goniometry, utilizing specified landmarks for any joint being assessed. This method meets the expectation of a standardized assessment; estimating, eyeballing, or labeling "WFL" does not. Documentation of range of motion should be specific to relevant joints and should reflect only those that were actually assessed. The focus should be on problem areas as indicated and how they impact specific functional tasks.

### Endurance

Endurance has become a dirty word in therapy circles based on the belief that its use will trigger a payment denial. The issue is not the term itself but rather in the fact that it has been used in documentation far too often. A classic example is an initial assessment that reads "Endurance: Fair" with a goal of "Endurance will be good." Moving from fair to good sounds like a measurable improvement, but key details are missing: What is that limited endurance preventing the patient from doing, and what will additional endurance mean for the patient's quality of life? Instead of addressing the core issue, many therapists simply avoid the word "endurance" and replace it with "activity tolerance." The situation has not improved in any real way when assessments now read "Activity tolerance: Fair" with a goal of "Activity tolerance will be good." The core issue is a lack of clear connection to meaningful information from the patient's perspective. OASIS item M1400 reflects this issue in the area of dyspnea, as the item asks for the level of activity that provokes shortness of breath not tied to any specific pulmonary diagnosis. Therapy assessments should look at the dyspnea component of activity as well.

## Edema

Circumferential measurements with consistent landmarks and specific descriptors such as pitting, combined with any impact on mobility, create a skilled assessment of edema beyond a "mild" or "moderate" designation.

## Cognition/communication/comprehension/psychosocial issues

Occupational therapists have a unique set of skills not only to assess these areas but also to directly tie any concerns to meaningful functional activities. Issues relevant to the occupational therapist's assessment include but are not limited to the following:

- ❑ Alertness
- ❑ Orientation
- ❑ Short-term memory
- ❑ Long-term memory
- ❑ Ability to follow one-step commands
- ❑ Ability to follow multiple-step commands
- ❑ Judgment
- ❑ Attention
- ❑ Receptive language skills
- ❑ Expressive language skills
- ❑ Depression
- ❑ Anxiety

### Environment

The home health occupational therapist understands the impact of the patient's environment on his or her ability to function. For example, kitchen appliances that are rather old and of questionable safety can add excitement to self-care training. Caring for a beloved pet is an IADL that the patient may care about more than any of the activities that he or she practiced in the facility prior to discharge. Family dynamics can add a whole new dimension to managing dressing and meal preparation, as roles in the home may be temporarily or permanently altered based on recent events. These factors are very real issues for the patient, and relevant information that is well documented supports the need for a skilled therapist to be involved with the plan of care.

 

### *Safety*

OASIS emphasizes the patient's safety when he or she is performing functional tasks. The challenge is defining safety in a way that is meaningful and specific to the patient. Simply calling something "safe" or "unsafe" is not sufficient; the factors that make a task safe versus unsafe must be included to reflect the skills of the therapist. Think about it this way: What is "safe" household management? First and foremost, that question does not contain any specific details about the task. For one patient, safety while doing laundry is maintained by having one person carry the clothes to the washing machine. Another patient may use her walker to transport the clothing but may need assistance to place them in the washing machine. A third may simply need cues to remember all of the steps involved in the correct order. The term "safe" does not stand alone as a measurement.

### *Sensorimotor*

As with the cognitive and communication category, a thorough occupational therapy assessment contains many relevant pieces of information that have direct bearing on meaningful functional tasks. Sensorimotor areas include but are not limited to the following:

- ❑ Vision
- ❑ Hearing
- ❑ Neglect
- ❑ Body scheme
- ❑ Motor planning
- ❑ Left/right discrimination
- ❑ Spatial relationships
- ❑ Discerning figure/ground

## Speech-Language Pathology

Utilization of speech-language pathology services in home health is directly affected by staffing availability. Many agencies have learned to live with limited access to this important discipline. Those that are in a unique situation with adequate or, dare I say, more than adequate staffing may find themselves under review because their practice patterns would differ from that of other home health providers. Overall volume of therapy visits is predominantly made up of physical therapy, followed by occupational therapy, with speech-language pathology making up a smaller percentage. This has nothing to do with importance or skill level, but it does put this specific therapy at a lower risk for targeted audit and denials, as there are fewer total cases to choose from.

The speech-language pathology assessment should cover more than just swallowing, and terms such as "impaired" without additional detail lack clarity about the true scope of the issue. Assessment areas include but are not limited to the following:

- ❑ Oral motor function
  - Strength, range of motion (ROM), sensation, and function
- ❑ Swallowing
  - Posture, positioning, consistencies, and diet
- ❑ Cognition
  - Attention, orientation, recall, and memory
- ❑ Speech/language
  - Articulation, comprehension, hearing, and expression

Therapy documentation needs to include information that is both measurable and meaningful. Anyone who reads a speech-language pathology assessment can become overwhelmed by the amount of measurable detail. There are often percentages, multiple and varied tests, and even the number of trials of gagging a patient with a frozen lemon glycerin swab. Of the three therapy disciplines, speech-language pathology generally outdoes the other two with respect to measurable information.

Remember, however, that the information must connect to activities that are meaningful to the patient. As an example, Mr. Phillips is currently able to recall a series of verbal items with 70% accuracy. However, without clarifying what the 30% deficit in performance means for his ability to manage his new medications or to communicate with his spouse, those numbers mean nothing. In contrast to how the assessment information was presented for physical and occupational therapy, the example will be of specific tool details to support the medical necessity of speech-language pathology. Record reviews reveal that the quality of the assessment is highly influenced by the content of the documentation tool provided for this discipline. Therefore, agencies would be wise to assess current and future tools to reduce the risk of denials by facilitating complete assessments.

 

Chapter 6

# Goals: Measurable and Meaningful

Just as therapy assessments create the foundation for the plan of care, goal statements provide a vision of the ultimate structure, and they guide the process of putting the building together. There is a common misconception that a set of therapy goals must include at least one specific statement related to strength, one for range of motion, and one for balance. In fact, there is no mandatory outline of goals that must be included for each therapy, and there is no template that will work for all home health patients.

Goals should meet two primary criteria: They should be measurable and they should be meaningful. This information is not new to therapists in any setting, and it is not specific to Medicare regulations. Keeping in mind the previous discussion of homebound status, goals must take into consideration the physical demands required to be mobile in the community. Setting high-level goals may negatively impact homebound status, but it creates the expectation of the level of function needed for patients to return to their lives. Once the goals are met, the patient would be considered no longer homebound.

## Measurable

Well-written goals correlate to assessment findings. The "measurement" component begins with collecting data consistently and incorporating relevant standardized tests as indicated. A deficit in strength, range of motion, or cognition does not necessitate skilled therapy interventions or always translate into the potential to improve, so more infor mation is required. Factors such as the length of time the patient has had the deficit and his or her willingness to work on improving the deficit are but two components of what is referred to as "rehabilitation potential" and must be considered when developing therapy goals. Goals must contain a measurement to reflect the impact of treatment on specific aspects of each unique patient's skills and abilities.

Periodic rumors arise surrounding the use of measurements, such as gait distances in physical therapy goals. The most common such rumor is that setting a target of more than 150 feet will lead to a denial of payment. However, there is nothing currently in the regulations resembling a list of specific distances that put a record at risk.

Measurements without meaning create incomplete goals, such as the following:

- "Patient will ambulate safely 200 feet"
  - "Safely" is not clearly defined with patient-specific details, such as equipment use and/or level of assistance needed.
  - Unable to determine what is important to the patient that requires 200 feet to access.
- "Patient will increase right shoulder ROM to WFL"
  - "ROM" is not defined in relevant terms of active or passive range of motion.
  - "WFL" does not connect range of motion to a meaningful functional task that will be improved by this "increase."
- "Increase speech intelligibility to 80%"
  - "Increase" would indicate some improvement, but the relevance of 80% is unclear.
  - "Intelligibility" is not connected to a specific meaningful task.

Pay attention to useful and clear measurements when creating goals, but such measurements do not stand alone in supporting the medical necessity of therapy services.

## Meaningful

Patients must actively engage in creating their plan of care and goals, and their engagement must be reflected in more than just the statement that "patient agrees with the plan of care." It is unlikely that a home health patient has actually stated the desire to "ambulate 200 feet with a walker and SBA." Rather, appropriate goals contain information that is relevant and important to the patient, and they put the therapy interventions into a meaningful context. It is possible to become too focused on the perception of functionality, as seen in these examples:

- "Patient will ambulate household distances with/without AD independently"
  - "Household" is not defined and varies greatly depending on living

 

situation. Without a standard definition, there is no clear way to determine when the goal is reached.
  - "With/without AD" is problematic; it should be one or the other with respect to use of an assistive device.

- "Patient will complete home management skills safely"
  - "Home management" is not task specific, and it is unclear which components are going to be addressed.
  - "Safely" is not a measurement and requires more patient-specific detail with respect to any equipment or level of assistance required.

- "Patient will demonstrate improved communication skills"
  - "Improved" sounds meaningful but is not clearly defined by an actual measurement.
  - "Communication skills" also sounds meaningful but is not specific in terms of components involved.

With the increased attention to the need for therapy goals to be meaningful, it is possible to shift too far in that direction and to omit measurable detail, thus decreasing the ability to support medical necessity.

## How Many and How Often?

Discussion of therapy goals often includes debate around two specific issues: the number of goals that should be in a plan of care and the frequency at which these goals should be addressed in subsequent visits. There is currently no regulation that dictates a minimum or maximum number of therapy goals. Some documentation tools, both paper and electronic, provide a long list of possible goals from which a therapist can choose. Such a list can inadvertently trigger therapists to choose more goals than are actually necessary and create the idea that there "has to be" a goal for areas such as strength, range of motion, and balance in every care plan. Solid therapy goals reflect a level of focus on issues specific to the given patient and must be driven by functional relevance. For those reasons, it would be better to have two or three well-constructed goal statements than a list of 10 that are incomplete or fundamentally irrelevant to the patient.

The frequency at which each goal is addressed has been influenced in part by documentation tools available to the home health industry. There are no regulations that set standards for frequency, as the plan of care should move forward based on the patient's needs and changes in his or her condition and functional ability. Not every goal has to be addressed on every visit. Think of it this way: We all had to crawl before we could walk. There will be activities that need to be addressed earlier in the course of care in order to progress to other activities. Ultimately, the documentation has to support "goals met" at the time of discharge or explain why one or more goals were "not met." The strategy of addressing every goal on every visit to ensure that nothing is missed along the way can lead to very repetitive documentation, and it can undermine the therapist's ability to show clearly how the patient is benefitting from the skilled care.

## Finding Balance

Therapy goals require a balance between measurement and meaning. Both physical therapy and speech-language pathology goals tend to include more precise measurements but may lack clear functional relevance. Supporting the functional relevance of goals should be patient-specific—such as linking all gait-related goals to accessing the mailbox—and not standardized. Occupational therapy goals have a strategic advantage with respect to the "meaningful" component, with tasks such as dressing, bathing, and meal preparation being routine parts of the assessment, but they often leave out measurements that show progress and support ultimate goal attainment.

Do not refer to activities of daily living (ADL) and instrumental ADLs (IADL) in groups as opposed to individual activities, as doing so misses an opportunity to enhance the quality of the goals. More is not always better. There are times when goals are selected that are not supported by the assessment or reflected in the planned interventions. The appropriate balance between measurable and meaningful requires and ultimately supports the skills of each specific therapy provided to the patient.

### *Goal examples*

The following examples illustrate what proper goal statements look like in various areas.

#### Physical therapy

- **Gait:** determine where the patient wants to go
  - ❑ Patient will ambulate 250 feet with walker independently on even and uneven surfaces to allow access to vehicle for transport from the home

 

- Patient will ambulate 1,000 feet with supervision to allow her to go grocery shopping with her granddaughter, as was her prior level of function

- **Transfers:** consider what the improvement will allow the patient to do
  - Patient will complete sit-to-stand transfer independently, pushing up from the armrests consistently to steady self
  - Patient will be able to get up from floor level with supervision as a fall recovery strategy
- **Bed mobility:** include impact on caregivers
  - Patient will perform bridging with 25% verbal cues to assist caregiver with hygiene and dressing
  - Patient will roll bilaterally independently using bed railings as needed
- **Fall risk:** connect specific risks addressed by physical therapy
  - Patient will remove throw rugs from living areas to decrease risk of tripping when ambulating with walker
  - Patient's son will provide supervision when ambulating outdoors to decrease risk of falls based on periodic fatigue
- **Self-care:** ability to ambulate and transfer should connect to functional tasks
  - Patient will ambulate 50 feet independently to access his bathroom for toileting
  - Patient will be independent with wheelchair propulsion to 75 feet over carpet to access kitchen area for meals
- **Balance:** connect changes to function
  - Tinetti score will be 22 or higher, indicating a minimal risk for falls
  - Single leg stance will be one minute to improve ability to ascend and descend steps in home to sleeping area
- **Strength:** use actual measurements and connect to function
  - Left LE dorsiflexors will be 4+/5 to improve toe clearance during swing phase of gait and decrease risk of tripping
  - Right knee extensors will be 4/5 to improve symmetrical step length during gait cycle
- **Muscle tone:** connect changes to functional tasks
  - Tone in left hamstrings will be normalized to increase knee AROM to WFL

 

- ❑ Tone in right plantar flexors will be normalized to improve heel strike and decrease fall risk while ambulating

- **Range of motion**: connect goniometry of specific joints to functional issues
  - ❑ Right knee flexion will be 100 degrees to allow for foot flat in seated position
  - ❑ Left knee extension will be to neutral to improve posture during standing and decrease c/o back pain
- **Endurance:** utilize dyspnea as indicated and connect to functional task
  - ❑ Patient will tolerate ambulation to 300 feet without symptoms of dyspnea to allow access to backyard to interact with her dog
  - ❑ Patient will ascend and descend five stairs independently without symptoms of dyspnea
- **Edema:** include functional impact
  - ❑ Edema will decrease in the left foot to allow for proper shoes to be worn when ambulating
  - ❑ Edema will decrease in the right knee to allow full AROM
- **Cognitive/behavioral:** consider impact on function
  - ❑ Patient will complete entire home program independently without anxiety being observed or reported
  - ❑ Patient will verbally recall total hip precautions independently; will require supervision to ensure compliance with same based on current level of memory issues
- **Communication/comprehension:** consider impact on meaningful tasks
  - ❑ Patient will complete HEP with occasional verbal cues from her caregiver to ensure quality of performance
  - ❑ Patient will demonstrate use of communication board as directed by the SLP to communicate needs during wheelchair mobility tasks
- **Environment:** focus on what is unique to the patient situation
  - ❑ Patient's daughter will remove throw rugs from the bathroom to prevent tripping with the walker when accessing the toilet
  - ❑ Patient will ambulate to 100 feet in the home independently with FWW over moderately thick carpeting without loss of balance

 

- **Safety:** determine what makes the task or activity "safe" or "unsafe"
  - ❑ Patient will ambulate to 400 feet safely with supervision and a cane on uneven surfaces to allow access to bus stop in front of home
  - ❑ Patient will transfer on and off the toilet independently with safe and consistent use of commode frame
- **Vision:** consider impact on function
  - ❑ Patient will ambulate to 150 feet around home obstacles independently using her walker to compensate for blindness in left eye
  - ❑ Patient will recall the need to turn on the lights in her home in the evenings to improve her ability to see potential trip hazards
- **Sensation:** connect to function
  - ❑ Patient will be independent visually inspecting bilateral feet for pressure areas after ambulating for longer than 10 minutes due to decreased sensation as part of diabetic management
  - ❑ Patient will independently recall the need to visually confirm foot placement on stairs due to issues with proprioception to decrease risk for falls

## Occupational therapy

### *ADLs:*

- **Grooming**
  - ❑ Patient will brush her hair independently while standing unsupported at the sink
  - ❑ Patient will complete brushing his teeth with verbal cues for sequencing as indicated due to dementia
- **Dressing**
  - ❑ Patient will complete lower body dressing independently following total hip precaution with use of a dressing stick
  - ❑ Patient will perform upper body dressing with intermittent moderate assistance for left arm only as she will be in a sling for the next two months
- **Bathing**
  - ❑ Patient will bathe independently with a shower chair in place
  - ❑ Patient will bathe independently in a stand-up shower utilizing a grab bar to steady self as needed

 

- **Toileting hygiene**
  - ❑ Patient will require supervision for clothing management during toileting due to right arm being immobilized
  - ❑ Patient will complete perianal hygiene independently without loss of balance
- **Medication management**
  - ❑ Patient will demonstrate adequate fine-motor skills to open medication bottles independently
  - ❑ Patient will set up pillbox independently and accurately
- **Feeding**
  - ❑ AROM of right arm will be WFL to allow patient to complete feeding independently
  - ❑ Grip strength of left hand will be WFL to allow her to adequately hold a fork or spoon during self-feeding

*IADLs:*

- **Meal preparation**
  - ❑ Patient will be able to reheat a plate of food in the microwave independently
  - ❑ Patient will independently transport a plate of food from the counter to the table while using her cane
- **Money management**
  - ❑ Patient will be able to locate her purse 80% of the time when asked by keeping it in one consistent location
  - ❑ Patient will require supervision during check writing to ensure accuracy
- **Household management**
  - ❑ Patient will be independent with laundry tasks, incorporating his walker correctly
  - ❑ Patient will wipe off the counter independently after meal prep activity without loss of balance
- **Functional mobility:** address mobility impact on ADLs and IADLs
  - ❑ Patient will follow through with gait instructions from PT during meal preparation activities

 

- ❑ Patient will require supervision when gathering her clothing items; once collected, she will be independent with the task of dressing

- **Transfers:** consider what improvement will mean to the patient
  - ❑ Patient will complete toilet transfer independently, decreasing the workload of the caregiver
  - ❑ Patient will complete tub transfer independently using a transfer bench consistently
- **Bed mobility:** consider impact on caregivers
  - ❑ Patient will complete bridging independently to assist with lower body dressing
  - ❑ Patient will be able to change position in bed independently to decrease risk of pressure ulcers
- **Fall risk:** connect specific risks to need for occupational therapy
  - ❑ Patient will demonstrate use of transfer bench during every bathing activity to decrease risk for falls
  - ❑ Patient will increase upper extremity strength to WFL to allow patient to push up from her chair instead of trying to pull up on walker to decrease risk for falls
- **Balance:** consider tests and movement with more specific ratings than "poor, fair, good" while connecting issues to function
  - ❑ Patient will be able to reach bilaterally to targets at varying distances in a seated position without loss of balance to improve ability to manage self-care from wheelchair level
  - ❑ Patient will stand independently unsupported for five minutes at the kitchen counter without loss of balance to allow participation in meal preparation
- **Strength:** use actual measurements and connect to function
  - ❑ Increase strength of right elbow flexion to 5/5 to increase ability to feed self
  - ❑ Increase strength of bilateral elbow extension to 5/5 to decrease assist needed for sit-to-stand transfer to supervision
- **Muscle tone:** consider the impact on functional ability
  - ❑ Flexor tone in right UE will be normalized to decrease assistance needed for dressing and writing
  - ❑ Flexor tone in the left hand will decrease to allow initiation of appropriate splinting for contracture management

- **Range of motion:** connect goniometry of specific joints to functional issues
  - ❑ Right shoulder flexion AROM to 100 degrees to increase ability to groom
  - ❑ Left wrist extension AROM to neutral to gain proper hand position when using the walker
- **Endurance:** utilize dyspnea as indicated and connect to functional task
  - ❑ Patient will complete bathing task using tub seat with one rest break of less than two minutes to manage dyspnea
  - ❑ Patient will complete dressing activities, incorporating pursed-lip breathing skills without cues
- **Edema:** include circumferential measurements, descriptors, and functional impact
  - ❑ Edema in left hand will decrease to allow for full AROM and improve functional use of the hand
  - ❑ Patient will be independent in use of lower extremity compression stockings as part of edema management program
- **Cognition/communication/comprehension/psychosocial issues:** connect concerns to functional tasks
  - ❑ Patient will be able to independently prepare a meal requiring 10–15 steps without cues
  - ❑ Patient will demonstrate independent use of a diary to manage medications
- **Environment:** focus on what is unique to the patient situation
  - ❑ Patient will keep a set of dishes at counter level to remove need to reach into cabinets or use a step stool to access needed items
  - ❑ Patient will use a nonslip mat outside her shower whenever she is bathing to decrease fall risk upon exit
- **Safety:** determine what makes the task or activity "safe" or "unsafe"
  - ❑ Patient will complete bathing independently and with good safety awareness as seen in consistent use of transfer bench and handheld shower
  - ❑ Patient will require supervision during meal preparation due to safety concerns when handling cutlery
- **Sensorimotor:** connect issues to functional tasks
  - ❑ Patient will be independent using a modified phone due to her hearing impairment

 

- ❑ Patient will be independent reading medication labels with use of magnifying glass

### Speech therapy

- **Oral motor function:** strength, range of motion, sensation, and function
    - ❑ Patient will demonstrate normal lip closure at rest, and drooling will be absent
    - ❑ Coordination of tongue movements will normalize during feeding to improve quality of the activity
- **Swallowing:** posture, positioning, consistencies, and diet
    - ❑ Patient will be independent, with nectar-consistency restrictions to decrease risk of aspiration
    - ❑ Patient will utilize appropriate chin tuck during swallowing with supervision and occasional verbal cues
- **Cognition:** attention, orientation, recall, and memory
    - ❑ Patient will recall three- to five-step commands independently, which will improve her ability to recall information provided by her medical team
    - ❑ Patient will demonstrate independent use of a calendar to keep track of appointments
- **Speech/language:** articulation, comprehension, hearing, and expression
    - ❑ Patient will demonstrate comprehension of complex written material, such as the information provided with her prescriptions, to promote safe medication management
    - ❑ Patient will be independent with communication board to make needs known and increase interaction with family members in social situations

## Managing Goals

Any discussion of therapy goals raises questions about the model that should be used. There is debate in home health about creating a single set of goals for the episode of therapy versus establishing short- and long-term goals. From a regulatory perspective, there is no required method to follow, which leaves the decision up to therapist. There are pros and cons associated with both options, as follows:

### *Long-term goals only*

- Seem easier to manage and ensure follow-through with only one set of goals in place
- Decrease risk of missing a date adjustment, as target is always the end of care
- Have a tendency to lack specific detail in order to cover a longer period of time
- Requires only infrequent updates over the course of care in response to patient progress or lack thereof

### *Short- and long-term goals*

- Create intermediate targets by which to measure progress along the course of care
- Provide an opportunity to modify as needed when dates are met or extensions are needed
- Can appear to be arbitrary stop points toward the long-term goals
- Create the risk of missing the dates specified in the short-term goals without careful monitoring of compliance

Do not take shortcuts with goals, as the end result is a set of goals that lack substance and fail to support the need for therapy. Without a clear vision of the ultimate outcomes from participation with any of the three therapy disciplines, the decision to end care can be left open to interpretation.

 

Chapter 7

# Planning Care: Putting the Pieces Together

If the assessment provides the foundation and the goals create the vision, then the connection between the two is the plan of care. There are essentially two components to this process: clinical decision-making with respect to the selection of interventions and writing orders for physician signature. Establishing the plan of care requires an analysis of the assessment findings, an understanding of rehabilitation potential, and the ability to put together the most appropriate set of skilled interventions to reach the desired goals.

Over time, therapists complete this task without too much thought, which can result in plans of care that appear to be essentially the same regardless of the patient's condition. This can also happen with setting frequency and duration of care as well as selecting interventions. However, it's important to avoid these pitfalls. Support for the medical necessity of physical therapy, occupational therapy, and speech-language pathology requires an effective continuum of information within the documentation, of which the plan of care and related orders are critical elements.

## Setting Frequency and Duration

Upon completion of the assessment, the therapist must determine the frequency and duration of care. In an ideal world, this decision is driven exclusively by the patient's need for skilled services, but the very real issue of staffing shortages often hinders such decisions. Many home health agencies report staffing issues to varying degrees for all three therapy disciplines. Even those that appear to be adequately staffed confirm that one vacation or maternity leave can upset the balance and affect their ability to cover patient visits.

Any discussion around setting frequency and duration for therapy services should include the use of ranges. Common examples are "two to three times per week for four weeks" and "one to two times per week for three to four weeks." First and foremost, check with the state in which the therapist is practicing to determine whether there are any specific restrictions against the use of ranges in physician orders.

If agency policy does not allow the use of ranges, staff will be held to the more restrictive standard upon state survey. Once any regulatory issues are cleared, carefully weigh the decision about whether to use ranges before moving forward. Note that, when ranges are used, the assumption is that the visits will be delivered at the high end of the range at all times, and that any reduction is based solely on patient issues. Ranges are not intended to accommodate staffing challenges such as therapist illness or vacation. Thus, any decrease in frequency or duration must be documented to show why it occurred.

Additionally, ranges are expected to be written narrowly, such as "one to two times per week for six weeks" as compared to "one to three times per week for four to six weeks." Wider ranges raise questions as to the amount of therapy that a patient truly needs. In the second example, it could be anywhere from four to 18 total visits. Based on these types of concerns, many agencies do not allow the use of ranges. There is nothing inherently wrong with ranges, but agencies that use them are advised to keep a close watch on how nurses and therapists use them.

In the absence of ranges, concerns can arise about compliance with a clearly defined frequency and duration. These concerns are rooted in the risk of providing visits without orders. The "extra visit" delivered based on a scheduling error or the arrival of a piece of equipment must have an attached order, or it will not be covered. This challenge is typically seen in relation to duration, as therapists have been given a directive to cover the entire 60-day certification period even if they only plan to see the patient for two weeks. Once again, there is no specific regulation supporting or refuting this practice, and if this practice is set in agency policy, there could be issues on the state survey if therapists do not comply with it. Therapists need to understand why the practice is in place and always keep in mind that the amount of therapy must be defended as medically necessary, even if there are orders in place for additional care.

Many agencies utilize the therapy frequency and duration orders to estimate the number of therapy visits for OASIS item M2200 on the start of care for the purposes of projecting payment for the episode. Recent assessment of this projection's accuracy is less than 25%, which means that the plan of care can and should change over time as patient need dictates. The clinical decision to extend care beyond the original plan or to discontinue earlier than expected because the patient no longer needs a therapist's skills must be supported by the physician's signed, written orders to confirm his or her involvement in the plan of care.

 

## Orders and Medical Necessity

Every agency has a group of patients that seem to get referred for any and all services by their well intentioned physicians. Family members can further complicate this situation by requesting orders for therapy despite there being no reasonable expectation for additional improvement in function. Therapists can find themselves in the difficult position of having a physician order in hand but a lack of clinical support for skilled services. In that case, therapists should attempt to explain the situation clearly to the patient, family, and physician. Even if all of these parties insist that the care is necessary, it is still the therapist's responsibility to determine whether skilled interventions are warranted. If they are not, then provision of services is not considered covered.

For a Medicare patient, use of the Home Health Advance Beneficiary Notice (HHABN) can be an effective and professional way to handle the situation. The notice outlines in writing that the home health agency is willing to provide specific services to the patient but does not believe that those services will be covered under the Medicare benefit. The agency informs the patient of the potential cost of the services and asks for a signature confirming that the patient agrees to assume financial responsibility should Medicare choose not to pay based on a noncoverage decision. This form often changes the patient's and family's perspective about what the patient "needs."

Communicate any decisions made to the ordering physician. Also note that, although medical necessity will not be supported solely by the presence of a physician's order, visits can be denied if no order is in place.

### *485 versus supplemental orders*

The level of detail in the orders sent to the physician for signature varies depending on whether a therapist completes the admission to the agency or he or she completes the discipline-specific assessment after the case has been opened. Often referred to as the "485," the plan of care generated at the time of admission or recertification is intended to be interdisciplinary and contains a defined set of information about the patient, including but not limited to biographical data, certification dates, physician information, diagnoses, homebound status, activity limitations, and frequency, duration, goals, and interventions for all ordered services.

If all assessments occur within the first few days of the episode, then the therapy specific information should be included in this form and sent for physician signature. If time has lapsed and the 485 has already been completed, then frequency, duration, goals, and interventions should be sent by each specific therapy to the ordering physician. It is routine practice to document "eval and treat" on the 485 as a placeholder for therapy services, but additional specific orders will have to be generated, as "eval and treat" will not cover a course of physical therapy, occupational therapy, or speech-language pathology.

When utilizing electronic documentation tools, it can be difficult to actually see these orders, as they are pulled together from various fields within the system. Therapists should periodically read through the orders that are generated as part of the admission process or the discipline-specific assessment to ensure that the documentation captures the necessary and relevant information.

## *Selecting interventions*

The word "intervention" is often used when discussing care plan development. The dictionary definition raises a very interesting concept that appears to have been lost along the way: "Intervention" is synonymous with "interference" or "disruption." It implies active participation by the clinician, not passive observation. The documentation must show what the therapist was doing that could not be done by someone else, as well as the patient's response to these interventions. When conducting a visit, does the therapist really embrace the concept of being disruptive? This does not mean being loud or causing problems, but rather teaching or demonstrating something to the patient that puts him or her on a different path. That process begins with selecting appropriate interventions.

The clinical decision-making component of establishing a care plan requires more than selecting a few standard items from a list. The three therapy disciplines are often connected to a specific set of patient problems:

1. Physical therapy: Addresses gait issues
2. Occupational therapy: Addresses activities of daily living (ADL) and instrumental ADL (IADL) issues
3. Speech-language pathology: Addresses communication and swallowing issues

A review of records indicates that all three therapies have become quite comfortable implementing a very similar set of interventions regardless of patient status. Here are the most commonly seen interventions:

 

- **Physical therapy:**
  - ❑ Gait training
  - ❑ Transfer training
  - ❑ Balance training
  - ❑ Therapeutic exercises
- **Occupational therapy**:
  - ❑ ADL retraining
  - ❑ IADL retraining
  - ❑ Therapeutic exercises
  - ❑ Energy conservation strategies
- **Speech-language pathology:**
  - ❑ Communication strategies
  - ❑ Oral motor training
  - ❑ Cognitive retraining
  - ❑ Memory strategies

Although some of the terminology may differ slightly, the general idea of what the terminology will look like is seen in the listed interventions. Electronic documentation tools often provide these as convenient options that are "point and click" and that generate the required information on the 485 or supplemental order without a second thought. However, establishing a plan of care that clearly supports the medical necessity of therapy services requires a second look at the words that are being chosen to make sure that the level of skill is clear. Consider these examples:

Mr. Max had a stroke about two weeks ago. His occupational therapist is going to provide "ADL retraining" per the written order. The actual plan is to address bathing issues that are complicated by the tone in his right arm.

Mrs. Bentley had an exacerbation of heart failure last week. Her occupational therapist is going to provide "ADL retraining" per the written order. The actual plan is to address toileting issues by implementing energy conservation strategies due to the dyspnea that limits her ability to perform this task on her own.

Mr. Stone has mild dementia and was recently started on three new medications. His occupational therapist is going to provide "ADL retraining" per the written order. The actual plan is to instruct him in the use of a pill planner to manage medications safely.

These examples demonstrate that terms such as "ADL retraining" may not communicate the level of skilled care being provided by occupational therapy. Similar issues are seen with the intervention of "gait training," as there are countless factors that can affect the ability to ambulate and that necessitate a patient-specific plan of action. Although there is nothing inherently incorrect about the interventions being listed in this way, it may be insufficient to establish medical necessity. The therapist should look back at the assessment for the issues identified, especially the "why" behind them, and customize interventions accordingly.

Examples of more detailed interventions for each of the three therapies are as follows. These are not meant to be a new list from which to generate information but are meant to provoke thought about what makes skilled care uniquely physical therapy, occupational therapy, or speech-language pathology in addressing unique patient issues.

### Physical therapy

- Gait training focused on balance and strength deficits
- Gait training incorporating compensatory strategies for visual deficits
- Transfer training: Sit-to-stand from recliner focused on pain limiting mobility
- Transfer training: On/off bedside commode focused on lower extremity (LE) weakness issues
- Balance training in standing, incorporating leg length discrepancy
- Balance training in standing, focused on vertigo and LE weakness

### Occupational therapy

- ADL retraining: Bathing inclusive of fear issue due to recent fall
- ADL retraining: Lower-body dressing using adaptive equipment
- ADL retraining: Grooming with focus on cognitive limitations
- IADL retraining: Laundry management incorporating use of new walker
- IADL retraining: Meal prep using microwave following multiple-step commands
- Energy conservation: Pursed-lip breathing during bathing activities

 

### Speech-language pathology

- Communication strategies: Focus on ability to communicate basic needs to caregivers
- Oral motor training: Focus on tongue coordination
- Oral motor training: Focus on improving the quality of the swallow function
- Cognitive retraining: Establish a drug diary for medication management
- Cognitive retraining: Focus on moving to mastery of multiple-step commands
- Memory strategies: Instruct in use of calendar to track appointments

Beyond the areas traditionally considered to be therapy related, a comprehensive care plan may also address interfering pain, pressure ulcer risk, and management of incontinence and skin integrity. Keep in mind that each individual service is one piece of the overall care plan for the patient. The most effective plans of care keep the patient at the center and are truly interdisciplinary, utilizing the full scope of skills available as a coordinated team.

Therapists often worry about the amount of information they need to document to provide enough detail; however, the examples provided show that it doesn't require multiple paragraphs to communicate detailed interventions clearly.

Chapter 8

# Routine Visits: The Need for Ongoing Therapy

In a comprehensive set of therapy documentation, from the initial assessment to ultimate discharge, there are certain time points that tend to reflect a higher level of content than others. Assessments are designed to include detail in support of skilled activities being done on a given visit. The same is generally true for therapy visits that are connected to completion of the OASIS, such as discharge from the agency. The breakdown in content that affects the therapist's ability to support medical necessity, however, is more often seen on a routine follow up visit. Therapists are challenged to remain focused on what constitutes skilled care and ensure that the quality of documentation is consistent throughout the episode.

Ask a group of therapists to complete the statement "Every visit must …" and it will often produce a chorus of "stand alone." This reflects a continued reliance on the concept that as long as "skill" is shown on every visit, then everything is in good shape. But how sturdy would the structure be if every brick was strong individually but had no connection to any other brick? The end result would be a pile of bricks instead of a solid building. There needs to be a relationship between visits that reflects the plan of care in action and there needs to be intentionality in every encounter with the patient.

## Continuity

When assessing the visit patterns of clinicians practicing in home health, all three therapy disciplines tend to have a higher level of continuity than does nursing. In many cases, there are only one or two individual physical therapists, occupational therapists, or speech-language pathologists working with the patient. Based on caseload demands, however, it is not unheard of for a patient to interact with five different nurses over the course of two weeks of care.

The risk involved with this lack of continuity is complacency with respect to documentation content. When there is a high likelihood that the same therapist will make most if not all of the subsequent visits, it is easy to miss aspects of documentation and to read between the lines when reviewing the notes, since the therapist knows the patient situation very well. As the total number of therapy visits increases, the quality of documentation content tends to decrease. The perception that therapy practice in home health has been influenced by the reimbursement structure of the prospective payment system calls into question the need for a higher number of therapy visits. Combining this concern with the aforementioned decline in documentation quality over time can be a recipe for denial. The issue raised is the need to remain focused on supporting the medical necessity of every therapy visit from the first one to the last.

## Defining Intervention

The term "intervention" is frequently used when developing care plans and supporting medical necessity on follow-up visits, but do we really understand what it means? According to Merriam-Webster's Medical Dictionary, intervention is "the act or fact or a method of interfering with the outcome or course especially of a condition or process (as to prevent harm or improve intervention)."

It is doubtful that any therapist has thought about the care he or she provides as "interfering," but that component is at the core of supporting skill. Therapy requires active participation of both the patient and the therapist. In addition, therapists must document clearly how the activities they choose are unique to one of the three therapies and could not have been done by someone else with the same results. Therapists generally do a good job demonstrating what the patient did during a visit, but they often leave themselves out of the picture. They often use statements such as the following:

- "Patient completed bathing activity"
- "Patient demonstrated dressing with adaptive equipment"
- "Patient progressed ambulation to 50 feet with walker"
- "Patient did home exercise program (HEP)"

The terms "completed," "demonstrated," "progressed," and "did" clearly indicate what the patient is doing during the activity but provide no clues as to what the therapist is doing other than recording observations. Referring to the therapist's actions during a visit as "gait training," "activities of daily living (ADL) retraining," or "oral motor training" does not offer enough detail. Those terms represent categories and do not convey the specifics of skilled care. The challenge, therefore, is to step out of old habits and plot a new course to demonstrate the value of therapy throughout an episode of care.

## Therapeutic Exercises

The area of therapeutic exercise provides a great example of both the lack of necessary detail and the opportunity to improve the quality of documentation content. Establishing an exercise program is routine for all three therapies and includes teaching the patient and/or caregiver how to follow through correctly. An exercise program is not intended to simply keep the patient occupied but rather is a prescription with a specific purpose. The myth that every patient must have an exercise program and that exercise must be part of every visit is just that—a myth.

Still, many patients do need such programs, and documentation of exercise is often viewed as tedious and redundant. It usually focuses on listing the specific exercise and number of repetitions associated with each. Statements such as "seated exercises × 10 reps," "standing exercises at sink × 15 reps," and "oral motor exercises × 10 reps" supply even less detail. Shortcuts such as "see exercises from last visit" are even more problematic. Although it is important to speak to the exercises themselves, there is a critical element missing: What is the therapist actually doing while exercises are being performed? If he or she is just counting, then the need for skilled intervention comes in question. Here are some examples:

- The physical therapist initiates standing hip abduction and hip extension exercises bilaterally as well as partial squats with Mr. Anderson on the third visit. Because this is new information, she has to demonstrate each of the exercises and provide continuous verbal cues to ensure proper performance. Confident that he understands the instructions, she leaves him with pictures to help him remember how to complete the exercises correctly. Her note indicates "the patient completed standing exercises at the counter × 10 reps each." On the next visit, Mr. Anderson proudly tells the physical therapist how well he did with his exercises, but when he starts to demonstrate, there are issues with his performance. He is not completing the full range of motion and tends to lean excessively during the hip exercises, but he does well with the squats. The therapist demonstrates the hip exercises again, and this time, the patient requires verbal cuing for about 50% of the task. On this visit, the therapist documents "the patient completed standing exercises at the counter × 10 reps each." Some

 

> may focus on the fact that each of the three exercises should have been listed, and they have a point, but the larger issue is that neither sample of the documentation reflects the demonstration or verbal cues provided by the therapist, as well as how those changed between the two visits, which are the components that actually demonstrate skilled care.

The occupational therapist instructs Mrs. Bond in an upper extremity exercise program using red theraband on the second visit, which is on a Friday. The therapist reviews written instructions including pictures, and with a few cues, Mrs. Bond is pleased with how well she can complete 10 repetitions. The therapist documents "patient performed UE ther ex with red theraband × 10 reps bilaterally." On Monday, Mrs. Bond's granddaughter is present for the visit and reports that the patient did so well that she had her do 15 repetitions without any increase in pain. When the therapist asks Mrs. Bond to demonstrate her program, he is very concerned that she is not anchoring the theraband correctly and not completing the full active range of motion as instructed. He asks the patient to find the pictures and goes over each exercise again step-by-step, including the granddaughter in the education. By the end of the visit, the occupational therapist is confident that they will be able to complete the exercises correctly but wants to check again on the next visit. For this visit, the therapist documents "patient performed UE ther ex with red theraband × 15 reps bilaterally." Although there is an increase in repetitions, there is no mention of the quality of performance or the skilled teaching provided by the therapist. In this example, the granddaughter was able to increase repetitions but did not notice the issues with technique. If progress with therapeutic exercises is only measured by repetitions, there is no need for skilled intervention by the occupational therapist.

The speech-language pathologist completes her assessment and, based on the findings, initiates an oral motor exercise program for Mr. Caldwell. She instructs him to perform these exercises in front of a mirror to make sure that he is doing them correctly and has his wife observe the session to provide reinforcement. Mr. Caldwell was recently diagnosed with dementia and has had some issues remembering new information. The therapist documents "patient instructed in oral motor exercises." On the next visit, the therapist notices that the mirror she had placed on the table was absent. When asked about it, the patient's wife reports that "it was in the way, so I moved it." After setting the mirror in place, the therapist asks the patient to complete the exercises. She is pleased that he is able to do them very well with respect to basic technique, but he hurries and does not complete the prescribed number of repetitions. The therapist reminds him to slow down and take his time. He reports, "I'm fine. I don't like these. Why do I have to do them?" The speech-language pathologist explains the purpose behind these exercises and how doing them will improve his ability to communicate clearly. He agrees that they are a good idea and slows down his performance. The therapist speaks with his wife about how the exercises should be performed as well. She documents "patient completed oral motor exercises." Not only is there a lack of detail as to the specific exercises and repetitions in the example, but the instruction provided is not captured at all. If the patient can "complete" these exercises without any issues noted, the need for a therapist to continue to observe him on future visits is not well supported.

Although including some form of exercise program is typically expected as part of a therapy plan of care, documentation connected to follow-up visits often omits the details that would confirm that the intervention requires the therapist's skills. This absence of information creates the impression that anyone can provide the same level of care. Therapists must not assume that documenting the name of an exercise along with the number of repetitions implies the complex level of skill that is actually involved in providing a therapeutic exercise program.

## Therapy and 'Training'

The plan of care sets the expectation of what will be addressed over the course of therapy. As mentioned earlier, the word "training" appears very often in therapy documentation; nursing's version of that word is "teaching." Based on many clinicians' documentation, it appears that they are visiting patients and training, training, training or teaching, teaching, and teaching over and over until the discharge visit. At that time, the patient suddenly learns everything and no longer needs training or teaching.

The problem is not with the word itself but with the context in which it is used. "Gait training," "ADL retraining," and "cognitive training" are not clearly defined terms. They should be seen as category headings that require additional patient-specific details. This is an extension of the discussion in the chapter on assessment: Documentation must connect to the specific deficits that are being addressed during the task.

- Mr. Dodds has Parkinson's disease. During gait training, the physical therapist assistant must cue him to take longer steps when using his walker and to be careful when moving from the linoleum to carpeting. She documents "Gait training: patient ambulated 75 feet × 1 with walker and standby assist (SBA)."

- ❑ Better option: Gait training: patient ambulated 75 feet × 1 with walker and SBA. He consistently requires verbal cues regarding step length and when transitioning surfaces.

- Mrs. Easton has heart failure and becomes short of breath when walking more than 20 feet. During gait training, the physical therapist assistant coaches her to perform her pursed-lip breathing when walking and to slow down her pace, as she tends to hurry. She documents "Gait training: patient ambulated 75 feet × 1 with walker and SBA."
  - ❑ Better option: Gait training: patient ambulated 75 feet × 1 with walker and SBA. She requires verbal cues to slow pace and was instructed in use of pursed-lip breathing when short of breath. 100% verbal cues needed for consistent follow-through.

- Mr. Finnegan had his hip replaced about two weeks ago and is anxious when putting weight on his right leg. During gait training, the physical therapist assistant encourages him not to stay up on his toes on the right foot anymore because his weight-bearing restriction was lifted. He is hesitant to try, but after the first few feet, he is able to put his foot down flat; however, he is still not putting much weight through it. She documents "Gait training: patient ambulated 75 feet × 1 with walker and SBA."
  - ❑ Better option: Gait training: patient ambulated 75 feet × 1 with walker and SBA. He requires consistent verbal cues for correct foot positioning on the right due to anxiety about recent change in weight-bearing status.

Training implies action. Suppose you decide to work with a personal trainer to meet your goals. The trainer arrives, takes a seat on your sofa, and begins to take notes. He asks you to demonstrate the exercises you have been doing up to this point and has no comments as you complete them. He tells you what a good job you did and proceeds to schedule the next appointment. Would you pay for this service? What is missing? The involvement of a trainer creates the expectation that he or she is going to do something that adds value to your current activity program. Critiquing performance, offering suggestions, adding new exercises, and pushing the program to new levels are implied in the word "trainer." If you could achieve the same results without the trainer, you would certainly not pay for this service. You will not reach your goals with passive observation alone and without the appropriate level of detail. It is the same with therapy documentation. Every visit must clearly show that what the therapist is contributing could not have been done by another discipline or by a nonskilled caregiver.

 

## Examples of Necessary Care

The following are a few examples of more detailed interventions for each of the three therapies. A single statement alone does not support medical necessity and must be integrated with other statements to create an accurate picture of the care provided to the patient. This list is not all-inclusive; the following are just a few examples to provoke thought about what makes skilled care uniquely physical therapy, occupational therapy, or speech-language pathology in addressing specific patient issues.

### Physical therapy

- **Gait training:** include more than distance, device, and level of assistance
  - ❑ Patient ambulated 50 feet with walker and minimal assistance due to weakness in left lower extremity and complaints of mild vertigo. Verbal cues required for 50% of the task for proper sequencing with the walker.
  - ❑ Patient ambulated 85 feet with cane and supervision on level surfaces and 25% verbal cues regarding cane placement. On grass in backyard, assistance increased to CGA and verbal cues to 50% due to increased unsteadiness, and distance decreased to 45 feet before rest break is needed.
- **Transfer training:** consider the components of each specific transfer
  - ❑ Patient required minimal assistance to scoot forward in her chair. Once in that position, she required SBA to complete a sit-to-stand transfer.
  - ❑ Patient instructed in pushing up from her chair using the armrests when coming to stand. He requires 100% verbal cues for this component due to limited attention span.
- **Bed mobility training:** outline challenges to specific aspects
  - ❑ Patient rolls to right with minimal assistance to reach railing due to pain limiting her ability to reach. Instructed her to reduce how far she attempts to reach to decrease level of pain during task.
  - ❑ Patient instructed in bridging to decrease the amount of assistance the caregiver has to provide during hygiene. Patient able to bridge with minimal assistance once feet are in place.
- **Fall risk reduction:** connect specific risks to need for physical therapy
  - ❑ Instructed patient and daughter to not use a step stool for reaching higher shelves due to recent fall.

- Patient wearing socks when ambulating and noted to slip slightly on the kitchen floor twice during gait training. Recommended the use of grip socks or nonskid slippers to reduce fall risk and patient agreeable. Will monitor for follow-through on subsequent visits.

- **Self-care training:** connect ability to ambulate and transfer to functional tasks
  - Patient ambulated 60 feet × 1 with rolling walker and minimal assistance, which increased to moderate assistance when going through doorway to access bathroom.
  - Patient ambulated up five steps to access her bedroom on second floor using railing and SBA due to fatigue after first two steps.
- **Balance training:** consider tests and movement with more specific ratings than "poor, fair, good"
  - Single leg stance: left = 20 seconds, right = 32 seconds.
  - Unsupported stance with eyes closed = 10 seconds with moderate increase in sway noted.
- **Strength training:** include the role of the therapist
  - Seated exercises: 10 reps each of hip flexion, knee extension, and ankle pumps bilaterally with 50% verbal cues to complete full AROM.
  - Standing exercises: 15 squats at counter with CGA due to increased unsteadiness as repetitions increase.
- **Muscle tone:** consider connection of tone to activity
  - Weight bearing through left hand on the armrest to assist with sit-to-stand transfer equalizes tone and increases ability to assist.
  - Weight shift in standing at counter with minimal assistance to right increasing weight bearing to decrease extensor tone in right leg.
- **Range of motion:** include the role of the therapist
  - AAROM of right knee extension × 10 repetitions with minimal assistance to achieve neutral.
  - Self-assisted PROM for left shoulder flexion × 10 reps with 75% verbal cues for correct technique.
- **Endurance training:** utilize dyspnea as indicated and connect to functional task
  - Progressing time patient can sustain ambulation this visit to three minutes before becoming SOB in preparation for cardiac rehab.

 

- ❑ Standing at side of bed for two minutes with minimal assistance × 2 with walker as pre-gait activity.

- **Edema management:** include circumferential measurements, descriptors, and functional impact
  - ❑ Upon arrival, noted that footrest was not near the patient's chair. It appears she has not been using it as instructed. Reviewed need to do so to decrease swelling in bilateral feet.
  - ❑ During ambulation noted that compression socks were not being worn. Patient's daughter reports they are being washed and she will put them back on this afternoon.
- **Cognitive/behavioral:** consider impact of plan of care
  - ❑ HEP instruction provided in picture format due to patient's inability to read.
  - ❑ Treatment session limited to 30 minutes as patient became anxious about visit to doctor later today.
- **Communication/comprehension:** consider impact of education
  - ❑ HEP instruction must be in written format for appropriate follow-through due to limited verbal comprehension.
  - ❑ Patient initiated use of communication board without reminders to tell therapist she wanted a drink. This was first instance of this noted with PT, indicating carryover of SLP instruction.
- **Environment:** focus on what is unique to the patient situation
  - ❑ Fatigue with ambulation is increased when on plush carpet in family room.
  - ❑ Patient requires minimal assistance with transfer from recliner chair due to low seat height. Patient unwilling to use a different chair or modify height of current chair.
- **Safety awareness:** determine what makes the task or activity "safe" or "unsafe"
  - ❑ Patient able to recall two of three hip precautions independently and verbal cues needed for no flexion past 90 degrees.
  - ❑ Patient requires verbal cues throughout tub transfer to maintain non-weight-bearing status of right lower extremity.
- **Vision:** consider impact on function and plan of care
  - ❑ Patient requires verbal cues to check for obstacles on the right side while ambulating due to limited peripheral vision in his right eye.

- ❑ HEP information converted to large print due to limited vision and improved carryover.

- **Sensation:** screen for problems that impact function as well as other issues
    - ❑ Instructed patient to visualize foot placement on stairs carefully due to peripheral neuropathy.
    - ❑ Patient required verbal reminder to inspect her feet after gait training with new slippers to check for any areas of pressure. She is a diabetic with decreased sensation in both feet.

## Occupational therapy

- **ADL retraining:** Focus on "why" the specific level of assistance is needed. ADLs include but are not limited to the following:
- **Grooming**
    - ❑ Patient completed shaving with supervision and verbal cues to complete multiple-step commands.
    - ❑ Patient requires minimal assistance to maintain balance while standing to brush hair.
- **Dressing**
    - ❑ Once clothing was handed to patient, minimal assistance needed to put on shirt due to left shoulder pain.
    - ❑ Patient requires moderate assistance with donning/doffing compression stocking due to decreased grip strength in left hand.
- **Bathing**
    - ❑ Instructed patient in correct placement of transfer bench and grab bars in preparation for shower training next week.
    - ❑ Patient requires maximum assistance with setup for sponge bathing and CGA during the task due to development of dyspnea after four minutes of activity.
- **Toileting hygiene**
    - ❑ Instructed the caregiver in how to support patient when leaning forward and provide minimal verbal cues to ensure that perineal hygiene is completed thoroughly.
    - ❑ Patient is able to use a dressing stick to pull up pants after using the toilet with SBA and occasional verbal cue for proper technique.

 

- **Medication management**
  - ❑ Practiced opening medication bottles with patient, who was able to complete task one of three attempts.
  - ❑ Pill planner color-coded and guide created to assist patient with keeping a.m. and p.m. medications separated correctly. Practiced using the guide with 50% verbal cues needed at this time.
- **Feeding**
  - ❑ Provided nonskid placemat to patient. With the plate secured she is able to feed herself independently.
  - ❑ Adapted spoon trialed with patient but did not improve his ability to feed himself. Will trial again in one week to allow strength to improve.

Instrumental activities of daily living (IADL) retraining: Focus on "why" the specific level of assistance is needed. IADLs include but are not limited to the following:

- **Meal preparation**
  - ❑ Walker tray delivered to patient over the weekend and attached by OTA correctly. Demonstrated to patient how to arrange items for transport in the kitchen. Currently she is not independent and will require supervision and occasional verbal cues to reinforce safe performance.
  - ❑ Discussed purchase of microwave with patient's son, as use of stove is currently unsafe due to leaving burners on when alone.
- **Money management**
  - ❑ Patient instructed how to organize incoming bills with colored files to improve ability to manage them herself. Currently she requires supervision with this task.
  - ❑ Patient now able to write with adapted pen independently. Applied this skill to simulated check writing and increased difficultly staying on specific lines due to visual issues. Provided additional simulated checks for patient to practice prior to next OT visit.
- **Household management**
  - ❑ Patient is currently dependent with laundry. Demonstrated the option of using a rolling basket to transport clothes. Patient able to return demo with SBA for balance.
  - ❑ Dishes arranged in cabinets to lower those used most often to within reach. Once completed, patient able to safely access dishes independently.

- **Functional mobility training:** address mobility impact on ADLs and IADLs
  - ❑ Reinforced use of walker when ambulating into bathroom for grooming activities.
  - ❑ Patient tends to leave her walker by the counter during meal preparation with increased unsteadiness when carrying items from the refrigerator to the stove.
- **Transfers training:** consider the components of each specific transfer
  - ❑ Patient completed shower transfer with supervision and reminders to use the grab bars.
  - ❑ Patient requires supervision when using the transfer bench due to memory issues with proper sequence. Instructed daughter how to assist patient and return demo confirms understanding of technique.
- **Bed mobility training:** outline challenges to specific aspects
  - ❑ Patient rolls to right with minimal assistance to reach railing due to pain limiting her ability to reach. Instructed her to reduce how far she attempts to reach to decrease level of pain during task.
  - ❑ Patient instructed in bridging to decrease the amount of assistance the caregiver has to provide during hygiene. Patient able to bridge with minimal assistance once feet are in place.
- **Fall risk reduction:** connect specific risks to need for occupational therapy
  - ❑ Instructed patient to remove throw rugs from the bathroom as walker gets caught on them during toileting. Patient verbalized understanding and will confirm follow-through on next visit.
  - ❑ Observation of dressing raises concerns over patient leaning too far over and leaning on the nightstand. Instructed patient in appropriate dressing technique using a reacher. Patient requires maximum verbal cues to complete.
- **Balance training:** consider tests and movement with more specific ratings than "poor, fair, good" while connecting issues to function
  - ❑ Reaching for objects outside base of support in sitting requires moderate assistance due to patient anxiety.
  - ❑ Static sitting at edge of bed requires CGA and tolerance is three minutes before pain limits continuation.

 

- **Strength training:** include the role of the therapist
  - ❑ Added 2 pounds of weight to shoulder flexion, abduction, and extension and decreased repetitions to 10 with supervision to ensure full range of motion is completed.
  - ❑ Review of HEP indicates patient is able to complete four of five exercises independently but requires verbal cues and demonstration to correctly complete full range of shoulder external rotation.
- **Muscle tone:** consider connection of tone to activity
  - ❑ Instructed caregiver in proper application of splint for right hand to decrease flexor tone in preparation for specific ADL tasks.
  - ❑ Patient requires maximum verbal cues to correctly complete stretching of right wrist as tone management strategy.
- **Range of motion:** include the role of the therapist
  - ❑ AAROM of right elbow extension × 10 repetitions with minimal assistance to achieve neutral.
  - ❑ Self-assisted PROM for left shoulder abduction × 10 reps with 75% verbal cues for correct technique.
- **Endurance training:** utilize dyspnea as indicated and connect to functional task
  - ❑ Patient able to complete bathing with CGA, requiring rest break after four minutes due to dyspnea.
  - ❑ Patient requires a seated rest break of three minutes during meal prep after completing 10 minutes of activity in standing.
  - ❑ During dressing, noted that compression socks were not being worn. Patient's daughter reports that they are being washed and she will put them back on this afternoon.
- **Edema:** include circumferential measurements, descriptors, and functional impact
  - ❑ Upon arrival, noted that footrest was not near the patient's chair. It appears she has not been using it as instructed. Reviewed need to do so to decrease swelling in bilateral feet.
  - ❑ During dressing noted that compression socks were not being worn. Patient's daughter reports they are being washed and she will put them back on this afternoon.

- **Cognition/communication/comprehension/psychosocial issues:** connect concerns to functional tasks
  - ❑ Patient requires 50% verbal cues to complete a five-step set of directions to reheat a meal.
  - ❑ Patient's HEP instructions provided in written form due to limited ability to comprehend verbal information. Patient able to return demo independently the three exercises communicated in this way and will confirm this strategy with the interdisciplinary team.
- **Environment**: focus on what is unique to the patient situation
  - ❑ Proximity of toilet to vanity prohibits use of commode frame, so training will utilize a raised toilet seat. Patient performs toilet transfer with supervision after setup and instruction.
  - ❑ Flooring in kitchen is uneven and impacts ability to smoothly roll a walker. Nonslip placemat added to walker tray to decrease slippage of items and patient instructed to utilize during meal preparation activities. Verbalized understanding this visit.
- **Safety:** determine what makes the task or activity "safe" or "unsafe"
  - ❑ Patient requires supervision during meal preparation due to impulsivity. Instructed caregiver how to verbally cue patient regarding pacing. Will need to reinforce compliance on next several visits.
  - ❑ Patient insisting on using a wooden board on his walker to transport items, which is not stable for larger items. Discussed trial with walker basket and he is willing to try this on next visit.
- **Sensorimotor:** connect issues to functional tasks
  - ❑ Instructed patient's new caregiver to increase volume when speaking with patient as he is not confused but is hearing impaired.
  - ❑ Patient requires minimal assistance during setup of medications due to vision limitations due to moderate macular degeneration. Compensatory strategies require 100% verbal cues to complete correctly at this time.

## Speech therapy

- **Oral motor function:** Strength, ROM, sensation, and function
  - ❑ Patient requires verbal cues 50% of the time with oral motor exercises involving his tongue for correct technique.

 

- ❑ Instructed patient on pacing breathing while speaking to manage impact of dyspnea. After demonstration of technique, patient able to return demo with minimal verbal cues.

- **Swallowing:** Posture, positioning, consistencies, and diet
  - ❑ Instructed caregiver in correct amount of thickener to achieve nectar consistency for beverages. Caregiver anxiety about this task leads to errors when he does not follow written instructions. Discussed the need to relax and make sure that the instructions are followed. Will need reinforcement on subsequent visits to confirm consistent follow-through.
  - ❑ Patient requires minimal assistance to achieve appropriate sitting posture when eating. As task progresses, verbal cues required to maintain position due to increasing fatigue.
- **Cognition/communication:** Attention, orientation, recall, and memory
  - ❑ Instructed patient's daughter to turn off the TV during meals to increase patient ability to focus on swallowing technique due to current level of distractibility and increasing risk of aspiration.
  - ❑ Patient provided with large-print calendar and with 100% verbal cues was able to write down home care appointments for the following week.
- **Speech/language:** Articulation, comprehension, hearing, and expression
  - ❑ Patient requires moderate verbal cues to decrease pace of verbal communication to improve ability to articulate clearly. Instructed caregiver in proper cueing for carryover until next visit.
  - ❑ Recommend visit to audiologist to assess effectiveness of current hearing aids. Provided a dry erase board to the patient and posted a sign to inform caregivers to write down information if patient is unable to hear them clearly.

## Fundamental Question

Novice and seasoned therapists can struggle to integrate themselves into their documentation on every visit, yet that integration supports the medical necessity of the care provided. In order to gain the proper perspective, ask yourself the following question when exiting the patient's home after the visit: What did I contribute that is unique to my discipline and indispensible to this particular patient?

Chapter 9

# Reassessments: Home Health Requirements

Assessments create the foundation for the plan of care, and reassessments act as periodic building inspections to make sure that everything is going as planned. The concept of reviewing the plan of care and determining whether modifications are needed was not created by Medicare and is not specific to home health. In fact, many therapy textbooks and published guidelines for practice present assessment and reassessment together as a unified concept. What is not defined in a universal standard, however, is when reassessments should occur. State practice acts and third party payers such as Medicare may step in and set time frames for any or all settings in which therapists practice.

For home health, there are two different mechanisms in place for formal review of the plan of care: recertification and reassessment. Both have documentation expectations that are rooted in the need to confirm that the care provided is medically necessary. If medical necessity is not clearly met, you risk denial of payment for services rendered.

## Therapy Reassessments

Although the recertification process applies to all home health services that plan to continue into another 60-day episode, mandatory reassessment is a specific requirement for therapy services that began in 2011. Practice patterns suggest that there are few patients who have therapy active at the time of recertification, as most therapy care plans begin and end within a single certification period. In those situations, there is no requirement to address when a therapy plan should be reviewed and updated.

Without any requirements, therapists were expected to complete the reassessment periodically and voluntarily to support the medical necessity of their services. However, there is little regularity with this task, even at time points where it is more obvious that such assessment is expected. Consider a case in which the speech-language pathologist evaluates a patient and the plan of care includes a frequency and duration of "2 times a week for 4 weeks." Initial goals and interventions are determined, and care delivery begins. Near the end of the fourth week, a new order appears that reads "Continue 2 week 2" with the same interventions as were listed on the original order. It seems that, on one of the visits made during the fourth week, the speech-language pathologist determined that additional care was needed. It could be that progress was slower than expected, there may have been cancelled visits that delayed attainment of goals, or perhaps progress was better than expected and new goals are being set. There was likely a clinical reason to extend care, yet far too often, little or no detail is documented. The visits in week four look like the ones completed in week three. Week five begins with no clear support for continuing care, and visits progress as though this was the original plan.

Although this approach may not affect the level of skilled care provided to the patient, the lack of documentation puts medical necessity at risk. Payer sources assume that, since more total therapy visits trigger more revenue, continued care with no clinical justification is likely driven more by financial implications than patient need. Medicare takes particular interest when the total number of therapy visits within a certification period reaches 14–19 or 20 or more, as those two points in the reimbursement continuum have the potential to add even more money to the episodic payment. In response to the lack of clarity and concerns regarding perceived incentives in the payment methodology, Medicare implemented the mandatory model for therapy reassessments, which affects episodes beginning on or after April 1, 2011.

## *Who is responsible?*

The task of completing the therapy reassessment falls to what Medicare calls the "qualified therapist" and not to the therapist assistant. The reasoning is that the skill set required to review the plan of care and to make changes based on clinical findings is within the scope of practice for the physical therapist, occupational therapist, and speech-language pathologist. Completion of the reassessment requires the qualified therapist to visit the home and should be incorporated into a treatment visit that is already planned for the patient. The reassessment requirement is not related in any way to supervisory visits for therapist assistants, and it is in effect for all home health agencies, including those that do not use assistants. The requirements currently apply to Medicare fee-for-service patients, but it will be important going forward to monitor expectations of other payment programs to ensure compliance.

 

## Components of reassessment

To understand the documentation expectation of a therapy reassessment, it is essential to be clear about the goal. To some therapists, use of the word "assessment" means that a complete new evaluation is required, while others believe that an OASIS form is somehow connected to this time point, but neither of these concepts is accurate. Rather, the intent of reassessment is to reevaluate the plan of care to confirm that the skilled therapy services continue to be warranted and to make changes as needed based on objective clinical information.

The following pieces of information must be clear in the documentation of a therapy reassessment visit:

1. **Objective assessments.** The data collected should relate back to the previous assessment to show measurable changes in the patient. Although it is not mandatory to include specific named tools, sequential measurements are important to quantify changes in the patient's functional status.
2. **Support for effectiveness of therapy.** "Effectiveness" is an interesting word choice, as it will not be enough to state "continue skilled physical therapy per plan of care." By definition, effectiveness is "producing a decided, decisive, claimed, or desired effect." Once again, therapists need to take credit for the complexity of the care that they provide from the first visit onward and must describe how those specific interventions affect the patient in a meaningful way.
3. **Plan to continue or discontinue services.** If the clinical findings and the therapist's professional judgment support a decision to continue or discontinue, the frequency and duration will be affected accordingly.
4. **New orders as indicated.** When changes to the plan of care are initiated, new orders for physician signature are to be generated in accordance with current regulations and agency policy.

For the purposes of tracking compliance, many agencies use a specific documentation form for the reassessment visits. Although there is no formal requirement to do so, the form can include triggers to ensure that the key components are present.

### *When are reassessments required?*

Most therapists agree that conducting reassessments is not a new concept and that the content requirements are reasonable to demonstrate ongoing medical necessity. The issue that causes greater frustration is the time points at which they must be completed.

Functional reassessments are required “minimally every 30 days,” regardless of the number of visits provided in that time period. There are two key concepts that must be understood to ensure that these visits are scheduled correctly: Tracking 30 days is driven by the calendar and is tied to each therapy separately. The specific therapy evaluation initiates the calendar day tracking for that specific discipline.

Each active therapy discipline must separately complete the reassessment. It is not within the scope of practice of one discipline to determine effectiveness and update the plan of care for another. As an example, the physical therapist can and should include information in the documentation that generally supports the need for occupational therapy services, but it cannot be responsible to create or update the plan of care—frequency/ duration, interventions, and goals—specific to that discipline.

### ‘Minimally every 30 days’

If the frequency and duration result in reaching 30 calendar days from the initial therapy assessment, then the reassessment is due prior to day 30. There is no definition of or time window connected to “minimally,” so the reassessment can be scheduled for week two or three of care when therapists anticipate reaching the 30-day requirement. Waiting until the last minute can create situations where reassessment visits are very close together or a patient cancellation risks noncompliance. When a reassessment is completed, the 30-day calendar is reset and the date of that visit is the next starting point.

- **Example:** The physical therapy plan of care is 2 week 6. A reassessment is anticipated at the end of the fourth week, but the therapist knows that the patient will be unavailable that week due to planned medical tests. Therefore, the therapist schedules the reassessment during week three at the same time as the supervisory visit for the physical therapy assistant.

## Exception Processes

Situations may arise that can impact therapists’ ability to complete reassessments at required time points. The key element in determining whether an exception process applies is whose responsibility the missed time point is. If a reassessment is missed due to lack of communication, a scheduling error, or an oversight on the part of agency or contract staff, the responsible party is the therapist/agency, and the exception processes would not apply. When a reassessment is missed due to circumstances outside the control of the therapist or agency, however, there are exception processes that can ensure that compliance is maintained. Consider the following examples.

 

### *Patient admitted to the inpatient setting*

If a patient is transferred to inpatient care, the agency will clearly provide no additional therapy visits during that time. If 30 calendar days lapse during the time when the patient was in the inpatient setting, the very first visit from any active therapy upon the patient's return should be conducted as a reassessment. Then compliance is maintained. No visits are lost in this process.

### *Patient cancelling therapy visits*

Patients will have bad days or conflicts with their schedules. When the patient cancels visits, those cancellations affect the cumulative count, especially in a multiple-therapy case. Each and every cancellation should be documented, along with clear reasons and acknowledgment of the impact on reassessment timing that was outside the therapist's control.

### *Natural disasters or emergencies*

When visits cannot be made as a result of natural disasters or other emergencies, the tracking of the calendar days does not stop. Once again, documentation is key, and reassessment must be completed as soon as possible.

### *Putting a patient on 'hold'*

When visits are stopped, the 30-day calendar does not stop. The decision to place a patient on "hold" is not random: Either the doctor ordered it, or the therapist evaluated the situation and used clear clinical reasoning to reach the decision. A well-documented note to support the decision to place the patient on hold meets the intent of a reassessment and resets the next 30-day window.

## What Happens When Reassessments Are Missed?

Therapists should make every effort to ensure compliance, both in the timing of the reassessment and in using skilled documentation to support medical necessity. Despite best efforts, there may be times when a reassessment is missed due to an oversight by the therapist or agency. In such an instance, there are implications for billing and reimbursement that come into play, and understanding the process will help everyone work toward continued compliance.

 

### *Nonbillable or noncovered*

Visits affected by a missed reassessment are deemed noncovered because an additional requirement was not met. Even though they are not payable, noncovered visits should be reported on the claim as a means of reporting cost and tracking the impact of missed reassessments. The term "nonbillable" should not be used in this situation, as that designation is attached to the level of skilled care seen on the visit. For example, sending a physical therapist and a physical therapist assistant to the home for a supervisory visit would result in only one visit that counts as billable. Although this debate may seem semantic, it is imperative that correct terminology be used in reporting these visits.

### *Missed reassessment visit = not covered*

If it is missed, the visit on which a reassessment was supposed to be completed will be considered noncovered. Consider the following example:

- The patient received an occupational therapy visit on days 24 and 28, but the reassessment was not completed until day 32. The visit on day 32 would be covered, but the one on day 28 will not, as it is the one on which the reassessment should have been completed.

### *Payment resumes 'on' a missed reassessment*

When a reassessment is late, payment is withheld, starting with the visit during which it was supposed to be conducted. Payment resumes only on the visit during which the reassessment is finally completed. Consider the following example:

- Physical therapy provides visits on days 28, 33, and 35 but does not complete the reassessment until day 38. The visit on day 28 is not covered because it is the one during which the reassessment should have been completed. Visits on days 33 and 35 are also not covered because the reassessment had still not been completed.

Despite the logistical issues, periodic reevaluation of the care plan to confirm the effectiveness of therapy in home health is an important component of supporting medical necessity. It is an opportunity to put the pieces together and to show the meaningful benefits to the patient, as well as to preserve the role of skilled therapy services in effective and efficient interdisciplinary care.

 

Chapter 10

# Tips for Qualified Therapists

The amount of information and regulations that the home health therapist must understand and manage can be overwhelming. Documentation issues can seem secondary to clinical concerns, but it is the delivery of efficient and effective care that ultimately creates documentation that clearly supports medical necessity. In an effort to promote improved focus and to move care forward, we've compiled the following important notes about key issues as they relate to qualified therapists.

| **Outcome and Assessment Information Set (OASIS)** |
|---|
| ❑ Completion of the OASIS tool is only one part of a comprehensive assessment at any time point—Start of Care, Resumption of Care, Recertification, Transfer, Other Follow-up, or Discharge. Include discipline- and agency-specific information to create a detailed skilled visit.<br>❑ Time the therapy assessment so that it creates the opportunity to provide collaborative information to improve the accuracy of OASIS data collection.<br>❑ OASIS items that affect outcomes and risk adjustment should be considered as components of a thorough therapy assessment and meaningful care plan, regardless of whether the therapist completes the OASIS tool. |
| **Assessments** |
| ❑ Objective measurements are integral to supporting medical necessity. Measurements must be taken in a standardized manner, and there are formal tools and tests available to help make that possible. In addition, analysis of testing results can support the need for skilled interventions.<br>❑ Connect identified deficits (such as muscle weakness or limited range of motion) to a functional task to address "why" those deficits are present. Assessments should include both the quantity and quality of performance.<br>❑ Factors that can impact the course of care, such as medication, visual, cognitive, or behavioral issues, should be noted in the assessment. |

| **Goals** |
|---|
| ❑ Goal statements must be measurable and meaningful. Functional relevance should be clear and specific.<br>❑ Goals related to activities of daily living and instrumental activities of daily living should be task specific and not treated as a group of activities.<br>❑ Goals must correlate to assessment findings and planned interventions. |
| **Planning Care** |
| ❑ Interventions should be specific to issues identified during the assessment.<br>❑ "Training" is a category of activities and requires more detail to show why intervention is necessary.<br>❑ Orders should be as specific as possible and updated as needed. |
| **Routine Visits** |
| ❑ Documentation should include what the therapist is contributing to the quality and quantity of patient performance. It should not read as repeated reassessments or observations of how a patient performs an activity.<br>❑ Be careful with documentation of therapeutic exercises. The documentation must show what the therapist is doing beyond counting repetitions.<br>❑ The term "teaching" risks appearing repetitive if there is insufficient detail as to what is taught, any complicating factors, and how well the patient and/or caregiver retains and implements information. |
| **Reassessments** |
| ❑ Recertifications and reassessments must be completed by the physical therapist, occupational therapist, or speech-language pathologist. They require an actual visit with the patient and are considered to be part of a treatment visit.<br>❑ Accurate timing requires the therapist to actively manage certification dates, calendar days, and visit counts.<br>❑ Reassessments focus on evaluating the plan of care to determine the effectiveness of therapy and making relevant changes to that plan based on clinical findings. |

 

## Supervision of Assistants

- ❑ Consider individual state requirements to be the minimum for regulatory compliance. The patient's condition determines the qualified therapist's level of involvement, which may need to be more frequent than dictated by a state's practice act.
- ❑ Supervision requires active communication and collaboration between the qualified therapist and the therapist assistant, and documentation should contain evidence of these specific activities.
- ❑ The qualified therapist is responsible for directing the plan of care. The decision to extend or discontinue the plan, in part or in its entirety, is an ongoing process throughout the episode and is based on objective assessments and clinical expertise. The presence of orders alone will not support medical necessity.

Chapter 11

# Tips for Therapist Assistants

As is true for qualified therapists, the amount of information and regulations that the home health therapist assistant must understand and manage can be overwhelming. Documentation issues can seem secondary to clinical concerns, but it is the delivery of efficient and effective care that ultimately creates documentation that clearly supports medical necessity. In an effort to promote improved focus and to move care forward, we've compiled the following important notes about key issues as they relate to therapist assistants.

### Outcome and Assessment Information Set (OASIS)

- ❑ Accuracy of OASIS data collection can be enhanced by collaboration and communication with therapist assistants, who need a basic working knowledge of the OASIS items.
- ❑ Management of incontinence, interfering pain, and dyspnea are just a few examples of connecting the care provided by the therapist assistant to OASIS information.
- ❑ Therapist assistants must have a working knowledge of outcomes and process measures in order to understand how the care delivered relates to these larger issues for home health.

### Assessments

- ❑ Information collected on the assessment must be communicated to the therapist assistant in a timely manner prior to the first visit that he or she is going to complete. Verbal as well as written communication to direct the plan of care is required for safe patient care that follows the plan as designed.
- ❑ Although the therapist assistant does not complete the formal assessment, feedback regarding the quality of the documentation provided in an assessment enhances the ability to defend medical necessity.
- ❑ The therapist assistant's documentation must include a level of assessment of the patient's progression toward goals using appropriate measures

## Goals

- ❑ On every visit, consider the goals and clarify how the interventions planned for that particular patient encounter relate to them.
- ❑ As the patient progresses toward goals, communicate with the qualified therapist to update those goals on a regular basis and not just on the scheduled supervisory visits.
- ❑ If it appears that a goal is not attainable, communicate with the qualified therapist in a timely manner to make any changes as indicated.

## Planning Care

- ❑ Provide feedback to the qualified therapist about the plan of care to help enhance the quality of documentation and support medical necessity.
- ❑ As the plan of care progresses, adding or removing interventions requires action by the qualified therapist after collaboration with the therapist assistant and shows clinical decision-making throughout the episode.
- ❑ Addition of modalities to the care plan requires a physician order and clear documentation that the qualified therapist directed this addition. Such additions may include use of heating pads and ice packs that the patient may already own.

## Routine Visits

- ❑ Documentation should include what the therapist assistant is contributing to impact the quality and quantity of patient performance and should not read as repeated reassessments or observations of patient performance of activity.
- ❑ Be careful with documentation of therapeutic exercises: The documentation must show what the therapist assistant is doing beyond counting repetitions.
- ❑ The term "teaching" risks appearing repetitive if there is insufficient detail as to what is taught, any complicating factors, and how well the patient and/or caregiver retains and implements information.

## Reassessments

- ❑ To time reassessments accurately, the therapist assistant must actively participate in managing certification dates, calendar days, and visit counts.
- ❑ Feedback from the therapist assistant on the content of the documentation generated by a reassessment visit will provide an internal audit opportunity to confirm compliance.
- ❑ The therapist assistant must follow changes to the care plan that result from the reassessment visit, and documentation should demonstrate consistency with those updates.

 

## Supervision of Assistants

- ❑ Consider individual state requirements to be the minimum for regulatory compliance. The patient's condition determines the qualified therapist's level of involvement, which may need to be more frequent than dictated by a state's practice act.
- ❑ Supervision requires active two-way communication and collaboration between the qualified therapist and the therapist assistant, and documentation should contain evidence of these specific activities.
- ❑ The qualified therapist is responsible for directing the plan of care. The decision to extend or discontinue the plan, in part or in its entirety, is an ongoing process throughout the episode and is based on objective assessments and clinical expertise. The presence of orders alone will not support medical necessity.